A History of American Medicine from the Colonial Period to the Early Twentieth Century

A History of American Medicine from the Colonial Period to the Early Twentieth Century

Luis H. Toledo-Pereyra

The Edwin Mellen Press
Lewiston•Queenston•Lampeter

Library of Congress Cataloging-in-Publication Data

Toledo-Pereyra, Luis H.
A history of American medicine from the Colonial Period to the early Twentieth Century / by Luis H. Toledo-Pereyra
p. cm.
Includes bibliographical references and index.
ISBN-13: 978-0-7734-5530-6
ISBN-10: 0-7734-5530-2
I. Title.

hors série.

A CIP catalog record for this book is available from the British Library.

Front cover: Pennsylvania Hospital. (Obtained from Packard FR. *History of Medicine in the United States*. Vol. 1. New York: Hafner Publishing Co.; 1963.)

The Edwin Mellen Press
Box 450
Lewiston, New York
USA 14092-0450

The Edwin Mellen Press
Box 67
Queenston, Ontario
CANADA L0S 1L0

The Edwin Mellen Press, Ltd.
Lampeter, Ceredigion, Wales
UNITED KINGDOM SA48 8LT

Printed in the United States of America

DEDICATION

To all history students interested in the inquisitive nature of the discipline. To all students seeking the advancement of the history of medicine. To future generations of medical scholars with the firm desire that they will encounter new worlds to uncover and new mysteries to unravel and who will have the intense necessity to tell the whole story. To every one of them.

TABLE OF CONTENTS

LIST OF ILLUSTRATIONS

PREFACE: WHY THIS BOOK?

It is not surprising to assume that every book written is important and sufficiently necessary in the writer's mind. This book is not an exception. I would like to believe that this work would be helpful not only to physicians interested in American medical history, but also to the historian interested in the medical events that shaped this nation. A third audience, and an important one, is the students at the various universities registering for undergraduate and graduate courses on the history of medicine as well as those attending medical schools here and around the world.

As the references inside this text will attest, this is not the first book written on the history of American medicine. Many books of extraordinary value have been written before. The books of Packard, Duffy, and Cassedy are just a few of them that come immediately to mind. I have frequently consulted all of them within the context of this book. Every one has provided me with great insight and knowledge in the understanding of the history of American medicine.

Why, then, is a new book on American medical history needed? A simple answer could be that new authors writing in established topics frequently present a new perspective that might be of interest to the field. In my case, the necessity for this book was borne from my experience in teaching the history of American medicine for fourteen years at Western Michigan University and the acute need I encountered in the majority of my students of having a concise volume that will reflect the teachings of the course. This book hopefully reflects the need for a current scholastic work in the classroom, but also for those who may want to find a source of discussion about this unique and special topic in history.

Our desire is to satisfy the curiosity of those seeking new avenues of discovery in the history of American medicine. Our intent is to stimulate inquiry by asking more questions to uncover appropriate answers in medical history. Our goal is to present the history of medicine as a robust discipline to the student interested in finding the development of this intellectual pursuit in the United States of America. We welcome new ideas generated from this work.

FOREWORD

This book has long been needed as a concise review of American medical history for college level, graduate, and medical students. Past personal experiences with teaching courses in medical history include the use of multiple texts, each differing according to the orientation of their author, such as the social aspects of medicine, history of medical education, or the history of women in medicine, among others. Although all of these topics are important, it is probably not realistic to expect that college students will read many texts, even if they can afford them. This single author textbook gives a balanced view of American medical history, written by a surgeon with doctoral training in the history of medicine, who has an earnest interest in the humanities, including especially art in medicine. In addition to use in a college level course in the history of American medicine, it will be helpful to beginning graduate students in the field, to give an overview of the topic, before starting specialization, and at a time they are particularly susceptible to the biases of their major professor. Furthermore, this work will also serve well the medical student with a special interest in the history of medicine, or as a textbook in those medical schools that have a history sequence in their medical humanities offerings.

The organization of the text runs from the colonial period into the early 20th century. It provides the student with insight into the influence of Europe, including especially England and Scotland, on early American practice and medical education. It then works through the impact of Jacksonian democracy on medicine and the development of various sects. The chapter on the Civil War is of particular value and takes advantage of recent scholarship in the area, demonstrating for example, that military medicine was not simply having the patient bite the bullet and drink some whisky as an anesthetic before an amputation, as commonly believed by many to this day. The principles of Lister in applying the new science of bacteriology to surgery and the German academic influence on the development of scientific medicine in the United States are given due regard in relation to their importance to medical education and care. Of special significance is an extensive chapter which brings together information on the entry of woman and African-Americans into the medical scene in the United States. This provides an excellent review as well as pointing out the relevant references sources for additional study in these areas. Finally, the importance of philanthropy in upgrading medical education is developed through a cogent discussion of its influence on the development of the Johns Hopkins medical school, the improvement of the older institutions and the meaning of the Flexner report. The synthesis of all these topics by an author with no particular axe to grind has resulted in a very readable and useful volume for a highly varied patronage.

Ralph C. Gordon, M.D., M.A.
Department of Pediatrics
Michigan State University
Kalamazoo Center for Medical Studies
Kalamazoo, Michigan

ACKNOWLEDGEMENTS

Two people were particularly important in offering counsel and support in the arduous writing of this book. Noted medical historian, Ralph C. Gordon, spent countless hours going over the manuscript, reviewing references, offering books to study, and analyzing new information over a long period of time. We had a great number of personal meetings and innumerable cups of coffee together. And, as if this would not have been enough, he took the time to write an excellent foreword for this book. Thanks for all, Ralph. And from the University of Minnesota, recognized medical historian, excellent teacher, and writer, Leonard G. Wilson, took all the time necessary to carefully review all aspects of the manuscript, from conceptualization to historical accuracy to English syntax. Thanks for everything, Dr. Wilson. All good elements encountered in this book are a clear response to their doubts and unique and outstanding suggestions. All errors in historical conception, interpretation, and writing are solely my responsibility. I sincerely appreciate their kind and generous support.

CHAPTER 1
EUROPEANS INVADE INDIAN AMERICA*

Grit and audacity stimulated Europeans to face the innumerable hardships of their rigorous transatlantic voyage in the seventeenth century. More than a century earlier, Spain and Portugal had shown to the English how this enterprise could be handsomely rewarded. The English monarchy recognized the importance of securing new lands and its vast resources for the crown. The English decided at this moment that the invasion and colonization of the unknown America were risks worth taking.

By the 1750s, the people of the initial thirteen colonies that would become the United States of America already had their own people with their own customs and lifestyle. The American Indians who inhabited this land prior to the arrival of Europeans in 1607 had their own medicine, rituals and spirituality. The first medical practitioners and treatments that occurred in what would become English America were Native American.

This section reviews the arrival of the English to America, the medical knowledge and practical treatments they brought with them, the status of Indian medicine, and the initial steps that began the medical amalgamation of these two incredibly diverse cultures.

Arrival of the English to America: First Permanent Settlement

Captain Christopher Newport commanded the first English expedition that set out to colonize the Virginia territory. His three ships, *Susan Constant, Godspeed* and *Discovery*, arrived in the Chesapeake Bay on April 26, 1607. In honor of King James who had financed the voyage, they named their new

---

* Partially published in the *Journal of Investigative Surgery,* 16:311-314, 2003, by Toledo SE and Toledo-Pereyra LH.

settlement Jamestown. The first colonists were not skilled in carpentry, construction, or agriculture, nor did they have medical knowledge regarding herbs and anatomy. They did not anticipate disease and sickness. They assumed that most medical problems would arise from hard physical labor or injury. They possessed little or no knowledge of infection, the spread of disease, or even how the body reacted to hot and humid climates. The first settlers were thus extremely ill-prepared for what they encountered in Jamestown in 1607. They were adventurers who had no experience in land cultivation, house construction, or other necessary skills for such an endeavor.

The long voyage from England had taken a toll on their supplies. Rations had to be reduced to a pint of wheat or barley a day. Sometimes for twenty-six weeks in the middle of the ocean, the colonist received highly undesirable rations. They suffered from starvation and nutritional diseases (scurvy, beriberi, and many others). The lack of fresh water haunted the colonists as well. The fort was situated back from the James River, but still very close to the ocean. Salt water would often push back the fresh water in the James. At high tide the James was an estuary, but at low tide it was "full of slime and filth which was the destruction of many of our men" (Quinn). The settlers sometimes suffered greatly from typhoid and dysentery.

As if lack of food and water were not enough, the new settlers also suffered from their first encounters with their new neighbors. When they first saw Native Americans, they thought the tribes had applied an artificial coloring to their skin. The brown color of the natives' skin was not referred to as red until after the seventeenth century. The colonists were unaware that they had settled in one of the most heavily populated Indian communities on the eastern seaboard. There were perhaps fourteen thousand Indians in the area belonging to the thirty-two tribes of the Powhatan people. They were led by chief Wahunsonacock, known to the colonists as Powhatan. The colonists stayed in their dwellings for fear of being attacked by the so called "savages." Within a few weeks of their arrival, an attack almost brought an end to the colony. One colonist was killed and many others wounded. Only the sound from the ship's cannons saved the colony total destruction.

With few provisions and sparse medical supplies, the settlers were forced to imitate the native peoples. Although the Natives were seen as uncivilized and uneducated, they had been living off the land for many years. Not until the colonies were firmly established were Indians considered not helpful to their cause. The first inhabitants of Jamestown lived beside and respected the Indians for their knowledge of the country. This is a key point when understanding the structure of the first permanent settlement.

Defining the Medical Scene

The first Jamestown inhabitants included no educated English physicians. They did include barber-surgeons, chirurgeons, apothecaries, midwives, and folk practitioners. This was not different from small towns in England. In Europe, educated doctors practiced medicine according to the teachings of the ancient Greek physicians Hippocrates and Galen. Galen was a surgeon and anatomist who used the ideas of the humors to explain the courses of diseases. He described the anatomy and function of many organs. His influence lasted through the Renaissance when all previous principles were challenged by the new way of conceiving and introducing the knowledge of medicine. Vesalius (1514-1564), Harvey (1578-1657), and a few others in Europe began discovering a new kind of medicine in the sixteenth century.

With poor lines of communication, New World medicine was isolated from its European counterpart. Educated physicians attempted to heal by bloodletting, bingeing, and purging in an attempt to balance the humors in the body. In America, such ideas of educated medicine were rarely used. Settlers learned from the Indians to look for medicinal plants to treat the sick and hunted for food. Although skeptical of Indian remedies, the settlers ultimately found that Indian treatments were better than no treatment at all.

One reason for the little medical knowledge prevalent in the early times of the colony was a lack of medical knowledge in general. Another was the inability to obtain an education—which did not exist in 1607—specifically dealing with medicine and treatments. Inevitably, early seventeenth-century Jamestown was influenced by both English heritage and the strong presence of Native American culture.

In the first year, the colonists suffered greatly, losing all but thirty-eight of the original one hundred and fifty. The settling of Jamestown represented more than what a human being could bear; as some historians have quite correctly put it, it had all the elements of a horror story. People in the settlement starved to death or contracted diseases that made them too weak to stand. The Indians had prevented the colonists from planting crops by forcing them to stay in the fort, and the food supply diminished fast. After eating all of the available animals, some of the colonists resorted to eating humans. An Indian who had been buried was disinterred and "boiled and stewed with roots and herbs...Some licked the blood which had fallen from their weak fellows." These settlers were desperate to survive. They knew that another ship would be coming soon, and they wanted only to save their strength until the day when food and help would finally reach them. For many that day never came!

John Smith was one of the young colonists who decided that the only way that they would be able to survive in the new colony was to have peace and trade with the Powhatan tribes. They had the Indian corn (maize) that the colonists needed to survive, and when the new ship came, the colonists would have supplies that they could trade with the Indians. From the Indians they learned also the herbs that could be used for medicines, the trails of the land, and how to plant food crops. The key to the colony's survival relied upon the Indians, however unwilling, to provide them with supplies.

Even after ships arrived with new recruits and supplies, death still raged rampant through Jamestown colony. In 1622, a surprise attack by the Indians took three hundred and forty-seven lives. The massacre hit plantations spread along seventy miles of the banks of the James River. The colonists, unfamiliar with the fighting techniques of the Indians, did not realize that swift retaliation might have warded off future attacks. There was no escape from the death and destruction caused by the attacks. The lack of surgeons made it difficult for those who were injured to survive. A total of six thousand people came to Jamestown between 1607 and 1624. By 1625 only a weak twelve hundred remained. Most deaths occurred within the first two years of a person's arrival. Those who survived usually did so because of their physical and mental abilities to adjust to the new environment. The Chesapeake Bay area had the highest death rate with totals close to fifty percent.

Native American Medicine and Medical Practices

North American Indians were content and clearly satisfied with their way of life before Europeans arrived. After English colonists arrived in 1607, American Indians began to experience increasing difficulty, to the point of being demoralized and unable to defend their soil. Unfortunately, the first American Indians did not possess writing that could describe their medicine. Through oral traditions, we have come to learn the characteristics of Indian tribes and towns. Diseases were not rampant among Native Americans. In general, the Indians had good health. Many of the infectious diseases were not present before Europeans stepped on North American soil. The settlement of North America by the first English settlers was achieved by a combination of force and disease. Diseases conquered much of North America for the English!

American Indians included many tribes with various means of providing for themselves. They have been divided into six geographical or cultural areas (including part of Mexico): 1) the Far North, including the Algonquin, Chippewa, and Ottawa; 2) the Eastern Woodlands, including the Chippewa, Iroquois, and Menominee; 3) the Plains, including the Cheyenne, Comanche, and Sioux; 4) the Northwest Coast, including the Chinook, Quileute, and Tsimshian; 5) the California Intermountain, including the Hupa, Karok, Mohave, Pomo, and Ute; and 6) the Southwest, including the Apache, Navajo, Papago, Pima, Pueblo (Acoma, Hopi, Taos, etc.), and Yaqui. The treatment of disease also varied amongst the tribes.

Before 1607, many European epidemic and endemic diseases were unknown to Indians living in North America. Indians had no particular problems with sanitation. Their eating habits and outdoor lifestyle left them free of many other maladies. The main medical complaints originated from injury, digestive disorders, and rheumatism. According to some European observers, North American Indians had good stature and healthy bodies.

"The practice of medicine among the Indians of the United States area prior to their contact with Europeans cannot be understood without some knowledge of their spiritual life and religious beliefs" (Stone). This spirituality was the basis of Native Americans' medical practices. Sickness and disease were derived, according to Indian beliefs, from spirits of the body that were angered or displeased. In every aspect of life, Indians believed that unseen powers and spirits guided them. North American Indian medicine was, therefore, a religious medicine where the spirits clearly dominated men and their health. European medical beliefs were not as openly spiritual. However, Stone, a noted student of Indian medicine, indicated that European medicine was "inextricably commingled with European demonology, theology, and philosophy." What made Native American practices different?

Indians believed the cure of disease was achieved through pleasing the offended deity; protection from the deity resulted from continual worship and pleasing of the god. Members of the Indian tribes used different ways to commune with the spirits; however, all agreed that the spirit must be pleased before healing would take place. Stone further explains Indian medicine: "it is obvious that medicine to the Indian was not only physical but spiritual; and was brought into play not only to cure disease but to advise, protect, and insure success in both the ordinary and the unusual events of life of the individual, the family, and the tribe."

Throughout these spiritual, religious, and medical rites, Indian medicine had mediators called medicine men. Medicine men, who had many names including conjure doctor and shaman, were used as guides through the spiritual world. The medicine man was a religious leader responsible for interceding with the reigning god on behalf of the patient and his or her diseases. The obligation and responsibility of healing was completely left to the medicine men. They were relied on to help achieve balance between nature and the tribe by using certain herbs and plants to maintain the health and well being of the people. The shaman learned the laws of natural and ecological relationships. No one else could take his position of benefactor and selected physician.

When disease occurred, the medicine man needed to plead with the spirit causing the problem. In approaching the spirit, the medicine man would utilize dances, chants, incantations, medicine bags, amulets, and whatever else was necessary to obtain pardon from the offended spirit. Herbs, concoctions, sucking, sprinkling, and other remedies could be used as associated treatments. On other occasions, the medicine man would have to ask for support from friendly spirits, who might intervene with the upset spirit. His duties also included preparing herbs and plants and administering them to the sick. In addition, the shaman used mortars and pestles to mix medicines, flint blades for cutting, hollow carved bones for injections, and drums and rattles for ceremony. All of the tools used by the medicine men were natural and possessed their own spiritual value.

The powerful element the shaman possessed was his special medicine bag, which contained magical herbs. The bags were usually made of cured animal skins and decorated with symbolic ornaments. These bags were priceless to the shaman; those who lost their bags were disgraced and thought to suffer terrible sickness. Besides curing sick individuals, the medicine man had other responsibilities that involved ceremonies and ritualistic practices. These practices they believed kept crops plentiful, tribes free of epidemics, and brought overall good fortune to all in the tribe.

While ritual played a significant role in Native American healing, there was also what has been called "rational therapy," based in the use of botanicals. Indigenous botanicals were used in conjunction with spiritual rituals to aid in the healing process. The plants were prepared according to Indian traditions. The Indians boiled them in water, then administered infusions orally or rectally. The amounts were often large, and not infrequently the effect would be strongly emetic or cathartic. The treatments would be, in any event, mystical and not empirical. Indian medicine could be summarized as:

Indian medicine = spiritual rituals + botanicals = healing.

In a completely different approach, European medicine could be summarized as:

European medicine = practice of Galenism = healing.

One of the best known examples of rational therapy was the use of White Willow tree (*Salix alba*). When ingested, it was converted to a compound similar to acetylsalicylic acid or aspirin. It was used to relieve the aches and pains of fevers or arthritis. The ashes of the tree could also be used to treat sore or failing eyes. The interior wood was often mashed and used as an antibiotic for cuts and skin lesions.

Lobelia (*Lobelia inflata),* also known as gagroot or purge weed, was also used by the Indians to cure ailments. When smoked, Lobelia caused the bronchial tubes to dilate and was used to treat asthma, bronchitis, and whooping cough. Lobelia also had a somewhat narcotic effect, altering the mental state and disrupting the nervous system.

The mayapple (*Podophyllum peltamum*), also known as the mandrake or wild lemon, is a remedy still used today to cure venereal warts. The Indians used it in this way. In 1787 it was re-discovered by a German physician, Johann David Schopf, who listed the cure in the 1808 edition of the Pharmacopoeia of the Massachusetts Medical Society. Currently more than two hundred native species of plants are listed in the Pharmacopoeia of the United States of America as having been used effectively by Indian tribes. These herbs and remedies can be considered the building blocks of modern pharmacology. For those of us who have visited modern American Indian reservations, it is not difficult to understand the emphasis placed by them on botanical modes of medical treatment. Plants and the spiritual continue to be a great part of the Indian medical world. As one looks at the role of botanicals in Indian medicine, Rothstein, author of *American Physicians in the Nineteenth Century*, reminds us that:

> The earliest Spanish explorers of Central and South America recognized the value of drugs used by the natives and soon began to export American medicinal plants to Europe and through Spain. By the seventeenth century, quantities of cinchona bark, sarsaparilla, coca leaves (the source of cocaine), and other drugs were being brought to Europe from South America. These drugs had a major impact on sixteenth- and seventeenth century European therapeutics.

Additionally, North American Indians were successful in dealing with trauma, including fractures, dislocations, wounds, and hemorrhage. They knew how to make splints for fractures or dislocations, to use bird down, moss, and other substances to stop bleeding, and to clean wounds with water and other herbal preparations. They gave excellent primary care to patients with these problems. The treatment of pain was another area of their dedicated attention. According to John Duffy, foremost historian of Indian medicine from Maryland and Louisiana, they relied upon sweat baths, warm poultices, massage, and aromatic fumigation for the control of various pains. Indian medicine in North America, then, was a religious adventure with some valid and practical approaches.

In American Indian communities, only a shaman could administer herbs to heal the sick, but even medicine men could learn a few things from the colonists. The colonists used one particular device to ease a variety of ailments. Alcohol would dull pain and make problems go away. When the Indians learned of whiskey and the effect it had on a person, they called it "medicine water." Some Indians used whiskey and rum to excess. Some, but not all, would trade furs for alcohol. Chief Powhatan would only take out the rum he was given as a present when the colonists were around. He never seemed to drink alone.

Differences Between Indian and English Medicine

English medicine that was brought to America, like that of the Indians, had no regard for critical experimentation, but paid attention to practical details and had a less religious approach. Despite this, at the time of the first English settlements in North America, their medicine was less effective than that practiced by many American Indian tribes. In fact, there was no universal therapeutic approach in Europe. Well-proven medications were almost non-existent. Despite dedicated effort, physicians would not find effective treatments for years, even centuries, to come. Patience and faith were the most important virtues that patients could possess.

Table 1.1: Differences Between American Indian and English Medicine at the Time of Colonization

	European Medicine	Indian Medicine*
Spiritual basis	Minimal to none	Yes
Religious influence	Minimal	Yes
Use of botanicals*	Minimal	Yes
Presence of infectious diseases, e.g. malaria, smallpox, typhus, etc.	Yes	No
Able in the management of trauma, dislocations, fractures, abrasions	Yes	Yes
Skilled in treating pains of neuralgia and rheumatism	Minimal	Yes
*Use dependant on spiritual basis more than empirical one.		

At the beginning of the seventeenth century, North American Indian medicine was appropriate for the care of the suffering Indian, and it was not too distant, in essence, from the best European medical practices. In years to come Indian medicine would remain stagnant while European and North American medicine would grow with science and understanding. This would eventually become a rational approach to diagnosis and treatment. Indians viewed disease as part of the total environment which included the individual, the community, the natural world, and the world of ancestors and spirits. Like the European teachings of the imbalance of the humors causing disease, the Indians believed that everything was balanced in the world. Imbalance caused disease for them as well. Other differences between traditional Indian medicine and orthodox European medicine would be the presence of empiricism versus no empiricism, the existence of rationalism versus spiritualism, and the lofty consideration of practicality versus spirituality (Table 1.1). Although it did not fully occur for hundreds of years, the colonists were on the path of establishing a rational approach to medicine. This would result in restructuring the practice of medicine. Indians began to communicate freely with the colonists. They showed the settlers trails and taught them the words that they used to describe various elements of common life: succotash, moccasin, squash, pumpkin, tobacco, tomahawk, etc. Both groups finally realized that they had to cooperate if they were to live in the same area. Not all of the fighting ended. Some tribes throughout America continued to feel threatened by the colonists. Many Native Americans, unfamiliar with the concept of land ownership, felt that land should be for everyone to use.

Diseases Affecting English Colonial America

Disease played a major part in the death rates of colonists and Indians alike. Smallpox, one of the most highly communicable diseases introduced from Europe, took its toll on the new nation. Highly contagious, the disease was transmitted by anyone or practically anything with which the affected person had come in contact. This disease killed millions of Indians in the northern, central, and southern regions of North America. Indians had never been exposed to such a virus and had no immunity to it. Squanto, a Pawtuxet Indian from Massachusetts, was kidnapped twice by the colonists. When he finally returned home, he found his entire tribe dead of disease. Inoculation, disease exposure under favorable and controlled circumstances, had not yet been discovered, and there was little hope for those who contracted the disease. Smallpox devastated colonial America with some of the worst outbreaks ever recorded. Between 1649 and 1792, Boston suffered from twelve epidemics. In one of the later outbreaks, when the town boasted eighteen thousand inhabitants, the only ones who did not suffer from the disease were those who had been previously affected and thus were immune.

Malaria, another disease that some scholars believe was brought to America by Europeans, also affected the populations of the new land. Malaria parasites were introduced in humans. The disease was disseminated by mosquitoes who fed on settlers arriving on infested ships from Europe. Since most of the plantations and villages were on or near the James River, mosquitoes possessed ample breeding grounds. The introduction of malaria confused the Indians, and they performed many rituals seeking understanding as to why their people were being punished with death.

The arrival of the English to Jamestown brought several infectious diseases not evident in America up to that time. These diseases annihilated an incredibly large proportion of the indigenous population. Smallpox, measles, tuberculosis, scarlet fever, diphtheria, typhoid, typhus, venereal diseases, and malaria were among the long list of diseases carried by the Europeans that infected the American Indians (Table 1.2). The dissemination of the microorganisms producing the infection was rapid and often fatal. No therapeutic armamentarium would become available until the twentieth century.

It is a sad irony that the English were the first to use germ warfare in the wars against the Indians. In Pontiac's Rebellion (1763-1764), General Jeffrey Amherst had suggested that Colonel Henry Bouquet distribute blankets filled with smallpox to the Indians. The disease was widely distributed among Indian camps, and death and devastation followed.

Table 1.2: Diseases that Pervaded English Colonial America

1. Starvation and nutritional diseases (scurvy, beriberi, etc.)
2. Malaria – brought in by English and Dutch vessels
3. Typhoid – generalized by European settlers
4. Influenza – serious effects in 1647 and 1683 in Virginia
5. Smallpox – the most dreadful disorder, came with European settlers, serious epidemics in 1630s, 1648-9, 1702, 1721, 1730-1, etc.
6. Yellow Fever – ravages of its effects from 1699-1702
7. Diphtheria – serious threats until 1735
8. Scarlet Fever – as diphtheria, serious threats in 1735
9. Diseases associated with bellyaches, cancers, bladder stones, flux, measles, and others.

The invasion of North America by the English and their diseases was devastating to the well-fed and healthy Indian nations, particularly when one realizes the lower incidence of disease in earlier times. Indians had no protective immune system for these unfamiliar European diseases. Thus, the Indian struggle remained centered around tolerance and survival. This was a fight that would continue for years – a fight of white and red, conquest and humiliation, control and imposition. It was a fight that would remain alive in the annals of European and American history for centuries.

Other Key Factors and First English Physician Settlers

At the time of the first Jamestown settlement in 1607, anatomy was the best known component of medicine. Trained doctors had knowledge of most of the structures of the human body. If they had read Andreas Vesalius' extraordinary work on human anatomy published in 1543, their knowledge would have been significantly advanced. Physiology had also begun its first steps in Europe. Other fundamental branches of medicine, as we know them today, did not yet exist. Treatments for disease were more harmful than helpful. "Without cities, hospitals, professional contacts, books, or instruments, the early colonial doctor acquired a resourcefulness, independence of action, courage, and ingenuity bred only in the school of necessity" (Blanton).

During the first eighteen years of settlement in Jamestown, medicine was provided to settlers through the London Company, a private enterprise made up of several companies including the East India Company and the Plymouth Company. Their main interest in Virginia was purely economical. A colony on the shores of Virginia might be expected to provide the mother country with trade it could always control. The company also had a commitment to providing the best medical care utilized in Europe up to that time. Many English physicians were interested in the colonization of Virginia and supported the London Company's project for a settlement. These interested physicians included Dr. Theodore Gulstone, Oxford graduate; Dr. Peter Turner, physician to Walter Raleigh; Dr. Leonard Poe, one of the king's doctors; Dr. Thomas Winston, a professor at Gresham College; and Dr. John Woodall, author of the book *Chirurgeon's Mate*. Woodall was concerned about the lack of milk in the colony and wanted to send cattle to it. These men were mindful of the need for medical expertise within the new colonies. Other members of the London Company also expressed interest in the affairs of the New World. Four years before the Jamestown settlement of 1607, Henry Keaton was the first English surgeon to land on the North American continent. He accompanied the fleet of Captain Bartholomew Gilbert, and while in the Chesapeake Bay, an Indian ambush terminated his life. Therefore, he was also the first English physician to perish while colonizing the new country and a hero to remember in English American history.

Colonial planters thought that more wounds and injuries would be caused by labor; therefore, two chirurgeons were to accompany the settlers: Will Wilkinson and Thomas Wotton. In *Medicine in Virginia in the Seventeenth Century*, author Wyndham Blanton states, "we have no record of Wilkinson other than inclusion of his name in the list of planters." Wilkinson was classed with the barbers of the time although the term "barber-surgeon" does not appear in Virginia records. The other was gentleman chirurgeon, Thomas Wotton. He came from a long line of prestigious medical practitioners in England, which included Edward and Henry Wotton. Wilkinson and Wotton were the entire medical force in Jamestown for the first eighteen months. In the summer of 1607, Captain John Smith credited the medical practices of Wotton for his own recovery along with the recovery of other soldiers. However, certain individuals did not agree with the medical practices of Wotton and refused Wotton needed resources.

In January of 1608, the next contingent of settlers reached Jamestown. They found only forty of the original colonists still alive. Among these forty, many were sick from unknown ailments. In the group of 120 settlers came four medical men: Dr. Walter Russel, physician, Post Ginnat, chirurgeon, and two apothecaries, Thomas Field and John Harford. Dr. Russel was the first educated physician to reach English America. There is no further mention of Post Ginnat or the two apothecaries; however, another man worked alongside Dr. Russel, Anthony Bagnall, a chirurgeon who accompanied Captain Smith on a number of excursions around Virginia. Bagnall was sought after more than Russel. Smith himself had wide experience as a surgeon and physician and had attended many patients before they sought attention from Dr. Russel. In 1609, however, a severe burn forced him to return to England because, according to him, there were no other chirurgeons in the fort. He did not return to America.

In 1610, Lord Delaware, the colonial governor, visited Virginia, bringing with him Dr. Lawrence Bohun, one of the most respected surgeons and physicians in the Netherlands. Americans praised Bohun for his extraordinary medical skills. A dwindling supply of medicines in Virginia stimulated Dr. Bohun to investigate the medicinal properties of native plants. He experimented with plants growing around Jamestown, including sassafras and another plant called *rubarbum album*. Dr. Bohun belonged to the humoral school because, placing great confidence "in the elements, fire, air, earth, water: the qualities hot, dry, moist, and cold: and the humors blood, phlegm, yellow and black bile" (Blanton). Sickness and disease meant an imbalance of humors within the body. Therefore, his treatments consisted of diaphoretics (sweating), purging, and substances that possessed alexipharmic (poison expelling) properties. In 1611, Dr. Bohun sailed with the governor of Virginia for Nevis in the West Indies. It is uncertain whether Dr. Bohun ever returned to Virginia, but while in Virginia, he was highly sought after for the treatment of medical problems. In 1620, the colony of Delaware named him Physician General. That same year, unfortunately, he was killed by a shot fired from a Spanish ship in the Caribbean.

The death of Dr. Bohun stimulated the London Company to send other well-trained physicians to the Virginia settlement. Dr. Gulstone recommended Dr. John Potts, who was well experienced in the art and practice of surgery and medicine. He arrived in 1621 and stayed in the colony until his death around 1642. Dr. Potts had an extraordinary apprentice, Richard Townsend, who excelled in medicine and surgery, as well as social and political affairs (Table 1.3).

Table 1.3. First Permanent Medical Settlers in English Colonial America

Year*	Type of Practice	Name
1607	Barber-Surgeon[Δ]	Will Wilkinson
	Chirurgeon	Thomas Wotton
1608	Physician	Dr. Walter Russel
	Chirurgeon	Post Ginnat
	Apothecary	Thomas Field
	Apothecary	John Hartford
	Chirurgeon	Anthony Bagnall
1610	Physician and Surgeon	Dr. Lawrence Bohun
1621	Surgeon and Physician	Dr. John Potts
	Potts's Apprentice	Richard Townsend

*In 1603, Henry Keaton was the first English surgeon to come to the area of Chesapeake Bay before a permanent settlement was sought.

[Δ] Surgeons were divided into: Barber-Surgeon (lowest type), Chirurgeon (had some kind of apprenticeship), and Gentleman Surgeon (educated professional).

Medical Education Amongst Jamestown Practitioners

The first educated physicians to practice in Virginia were selected and sent by the London Company. Their medical educations had been obtained like that of other well-educated English physicians of the day, at Oxford and Cambridge; however, better opportunities existed in Italy and France. A seventeenth-century English medical student would have been exposed to chemistry and physics. Clinical observation as a systematic way of teaching in Europe was just beginning to be introduced in medicine, but no instruction was given to students as to how to make appropriate and effective observations. Only apprenticeship offered a better means of becoming acquainted with the clinical practice of the day. Frequently, only wealthy individuals were able to study medicine formally and obtain medical degrees from universities. Blanton, historian of early American medicine, described the training of English physicians of the early seventeenth century: "The great majority of English physicians had had no university training. They were ordinary physicians, trained by apprenticeship: the chirurgeons, products sometimes of the Barbers-College, the bone settlers and others." Most medical men entered the field through an apprenticeship, which was not necessarily the best way to gain theoretical medical knowledge. Apprenticeships required working along side an established practitioner for usually six to eight years although apprenticeships could be as brief as one year. The London Company had planned to establish a number of free schools to provide medical training for colonial students, but funds for such schools were hard to come by, and the idea was given up only a year later. Most individuals gained medical knowledge in their homes. At that time it was possible for a few learned settlers to educate themselves by reading medical texts at home. In Virginia it is fair to say that only one-half of the population was literate. Little emphasis was put upon reading and writing in seventeenth-century Virginia. Rather, stress was placed on food production and overall good health.

A great many factors influenced life in Jamestown between 1607 and 1620. The first settlers' knowledge of medicine, agriculture, and life played an important part in their survival. Another influencing factor was the presence of the Native Americans, their different beliefs, and contrasting medical practices. Extremely different cultures, in close proximity in the same country, caused a great deal of tension, while at the same time allowing for a growing respect and the sharing of knowledge between them. Limited medical knowledge was the most influential factor in early Jamestown. In summary, the lack of schools and universities within the colonies was the main reason contributing to the severe absence of educated physicians within Virginia. Many of the practitioners of early Virginia were either of the apprentice type or just educated individuals trying to make a difference. Very few individuals had the money necessary to obtain medical education in Europe. Overall, medical knowledge and the opportunities to obtain this knowledge were extremely poor.

Conclusion

Indian medicine was the first medicine practiced on the American continent. English colonists who settled in Indian America brought a different but certainly not superior medical system. A number of barber-surgeons, chirurgeons, apothecaries, mid-wives, and a wide range of folk practitioners who came and left during the first years of English colonial America had minimal medical knowledge. They brought from England limited theoretical information, few practical considerations, and the unsettled intention to improve their unsophisticated methods. Indian Americans were content with their way of living and their health. The English invaded their country and brought with them disease and death. The Indian environment would be forever modified. English settlers brought diseases such as smallpox, malaria, and measles. Yellow fever came from Africa with the importation of Negro slaves. Systematic medical science was absent in the colonies for at least the first century of colonization. Colonial governors, clerics (minister-physicians), and self-educated practitioners provided medical care. Very seldom were physicians with formal education from well-respected European medical schools present in early colonial America. Clearly, the state of medicine in the early- and mid-1600s introduced by the English to the new colonies was not the best because the best was not yet available. Native Americans had a better approach to health and disease. Spiritual and botanical medicine was prevalent in the American Indian population. Even though North American Indians and Europeans unintentionally helped each other in the care of patients, little progress was garnered in the pioneering days of the colonies.

CHAPTER 2
COLONISTS IMPOSE THEMSELVES

As time passed in the thirteen colonies, the way of life and character of the inhabitants of the newly discovered land changed. It would take more than fifty years after the permanent settlement at Jamestown in 1607 before English colonists began to affect their new home and its environment decisively. Medical historian John Duffy identified the situation of colonial English America at the time:

> By 1700 the British foothold on the American continent was well established. The struggling settlements in New England and Virginia were becoming prosperous towns and communities, reproducing in part the social structure of the mother country...Those young colonials interested in medicine turned first to the British and European medical schools; then, as a consciousness of American nationality began to develop and American communities became large enough to support medical institutions, hospitals and medical schools made their appearance. By the time of the Revolution one hospital and two medical schools were firmly established, a number of local medical societies were functioning, and several colonies had enacted medical licensure laws.

This chapter continues the analysis of English American colonial medicine as it pertains to medical theories, the practice of medicine, the status of physicians here and abroad, medical education, and the laws regulating colonial physicians. Other notable medical practitioners, the introduction of inoculation, the review of certain diseases and medical treatments, and the development of general hospitals in the colonies complete this section.

More About English American Colonial Medicine

To understand English American colonial medicine, one must understand the times and circumstances in the colonies as well as the world as a whole. By the beginning of the seventeenth century, Europeans had begun to better understand anatomy through the extraordinary works of Andreas Vesalius (1514-1564). William Harvey's (1578-1657) magnificent concepts on the circulation of the blood began to be propagated and students started to become aware of them. These discoveries, however, meant little to the world at the time and considerably less to colonial America.

The first English physicians arrived in America much before the introduction of the innovative and revolutionary thinking of Thomas Sydenham (1624-1689) and Herman Boerhaave (1608-1738). Medical information was not widely distributed, and even if it were, little notice would have been made of it because no one had applied this knowledge to treat patients medically. Physics, chemistry, and medicine had not effectively intertwined as of yet. Early seventeenth century English physicians had little understanding of physiology or disease processes, and they had few efficacious medical treatments available. They were still practicing ancient Greek humoral medicine. The germ theory of disease was not recognized. Every physician, quack, and irregular scientist had his own theory about the human body and disease.

In the American colonies, the lack of information was exacerbated by the time it took for the few new publications to get to the New World. The lack of an educational system, hospitals, and medical schools, as well as the minimal amount of equipment or medications resulted in mediocre health care. During this period, the average life span in the colonies was 35 years. Only high birth rates kept the colonists' population from dwindling, with the average woman bearing seven children.

Jamestown received a large number of tired and diseased English individuals who had traveled for months and needed to survive the effects of the cruel voyage. Poor diet and dismal health resulted. All diseases, from nutritional to infectious problems, affected the debilitated English colonists. Treatments were not available or known at this time. The final outcome depended especially on the tolerance of the arriving individuals to the extraordinarily disgusting sanitary conditions present in the traveling ships.

At their arrival, Europeans expected to undergo seasoning. Seasoning meant the acquisition of some degree of immunity after reaching this country. Seasoning was necessary to survive the wide range of diseases and fevers the first year in Virginia. Eighty percent of colonists arriving between 1607 and 1625, or

4,800 out of 6,000, died from such diseases as fluxes, fevers, bellyaches, bloody flux, and malaria. When the first New England settlers arrived in Plymouth in 1620, they were able to profit from the early experience of the Virginians. Nevertheless, the pilgrims had to endure their own seasoning. During the first winter, almost half of the Plymouth colonists died.

Medical Theory and Practice

The major medical theory in the seventeenth century was based on the teachings of Galen (129-199 AD). Galenism was the basis for the medical practice of English physicians who came to the colonies. Galen considered that the body was ruled by four humors which determined both personality and reaction to different types of disease. The four humors were blood (a fiery personality), phlegm (a calm personality), yellow bile (a bad-tempered personality), and black bile (a melancholic personality). The qualities of these respective humors were hot, cold, moist, and dry (Table 2.1). For health, the humors had to remain in a state of balance. If a particular humor were in excess or deficiency, the physician would attempt to restore the body to its natural state. To do this, he used purging and bleeding.

Table 2.1. Basis of Galenism in the Practice of Western Medicine

Humors	Manifested Qualities
Yellow bile	Cold
Blood	Heat
Phlegm	Moistness
Black bile	Dryness

Imbalance of humors = disease
Treatment required balancing the humors

The presence of fever required a cooling regimen and sometimes bleeding to eliminate increased heat, chills required warm preparations, and dark stools required enemas or laxatives. Within the theories of Hippocratic teachings, physicians recommended appropriate diet, frequent exercise, and allowing nature to exercise its healing power. The sixteenth-century physician Paracelsus (1493-1541) used mineral or chemical remedies such as mercury, sulfur, iron, arsenic, copper, or potassium. Thomas Sydenham (1624-1689) reasserted the principles of Hippocrates; moderation was the essence of treatment as well as reliance upon the healing power of nature.

The practice of American colonial physicians was based on a modified humoral system, with the use of bleeding, blistering, purging, vomiting, and sweating. It continued until the mid-1800s. As William Douglass, a Boston, Massachusetts physician of the 1700s, educated at the University of Edinburgh, wrote, the treatment system in New England "was very uniform, bleeding, vomiting, blistering, purging, anodyne, etc. If the illness continued there was repetendi, and finally murderandi."

In the Colonial era, medical practitioners were few. Few physicians from England were willing to abandon their already established practices in the big cities to face the unknown of a new land. They generally preferred to live in a city where everything was established and life was easier. What reason had they to go to a pioneer society and face a harrowing sea voyage and an increased chance of disease? Because of this reluctance, there were few physicians coming to the English colonies. In America, medical practitioners might also be farmers, shopkeepers, or might hold other types of jobs. Medicine was not a full-time profession.

In 1620, the *Mayflower* brought several medical practitioners. Samuel Fuller, a minister-physician, had studied some medicine in London, where he may have had an apprenticeship. He also may have attended medical lectures in Leyden, where he worked part time as a weaver. The ship's log lists him as being a physician, surgeon, and doctor. The other doctor aboard was Giles Heale, the ship's surgeon. His training consisted of an apprenticeship and a license to practice issued by the Barber-Surgeons Company of London. Giles remained in Plymouth for only four months before returning to England.

Status of Physicians in England and the Colonies

English medical practitioners belonged to three distinct groups: apothecaries or druggists, surgeons, and physicians. Very few came to the New World. They were respected and had established practices. It was not worth the risk of dying on the trip when they were quite comfortable in England. Following this well-reasoned equation, most of the wealthy did not emigrate. The distinction between medicine, surgery, and pharmacy did not exist in colonial America. Out of necessity, American medical practitioners had to perform their own surgeries and mix their own medicines.

Surgery was generally performed to treat injury. It was a surgeon's job to control hemorrhage, close wounds, and repair dislocations and fractures. In the case of internal injuries, the patient was usually written off. Surgeons were generally less educated than physicians and tended to work in guilds. These guilds were where they learned their craft and existed as a way to control and regulate their profession.

University-educated physicians were few in the colonies. Practically anyone with any medical training whatsoever assumed the title of doctor. Of the 1,600 proclaimed doctors who practiced medicine in Massachusetts between the founding of Plymouth and the year of 1800, fewer than 100 were immigrants. American physicians were trained by apprenticeship if at all. Most of the immigrant practitioners came from Great Britain. Only about one-quarter of them received some form of medical training before arriving in the New World. Four of these people actually had MDs, eight attended a university of some sort, and thirteen of them gained experience in the armed forces. Among 1,370 medical practitioners in Massachusetts in the 18th century, only 399 attended college, and only 360 achieved a BA degree. Before 1700, even fewer Massachusetts physicians attended college.

Apprenticeship was the main mode of education. Anyone who could read and write was eligible to receive training. Students needed to seek a practitioner with whom they could study. A few students went to the newly-formed colonial colleges such as Harvard, and still fewer, such as Samuel Bellingham and John Glover, went to Europe to complete their medical educations before returning home to practice medicine.

Medical Education in England and English America

If a student chose to study medicine in England, he would most likely go to either Oxford or Cambridge, but these schools were available only to members of the Church of England. They granted medical diplomas after 14 years of attendance. To obtain a medical degree from one of these universities, one first had to earn a bachelor of arts, master of arts, and bachelor of medicine before being allowed to earn a medical doctorate. The training at these universities was mainly theoretical, with little or no practical experience. The student read the writings of the ancients and medieval commentaries on these ancient writers.

At Oxford and Cambridge Universities, the student had to study for six years, attend two dissections, participate in two debates and pass an exam to receive the Bachelor of Medicine degree. After two further disputations, dissections, and another exam, the student received a Medical Doctorate. To receive the Doctorate, the student was required to attend lectures given by the Regius Professor and to give six lectures on Galen or three cursory lectures on one of Galen's books, which include *Temperaments*, *Fevers*, *Parts*, and *Local Affections*. These were just the requirements to graduate from the university. To earn a license to practice medicine, the student also had to show three proven cures. After all this work, the new doctor could finally practice medicine.

The most celebrated European medical school in the late-colonial era was Edinburgh. Between 1749 and 1800, many colonists from the New World attended Edinburgh: 49 from Virginia, 16 from South Carolina, 15 from Pennsylvania, 10 from New York, 8 from Maryland, 3 from Georgia, 2 from Massachusetts. Not every student who went to Edinburgh received a MD degree. Most just attended lectures and did not receive a degree. Many students went to Edinburgh to study with a local physician. The letter of recommendation from this local doctor would serve as a diploma in unsophisticated colonial America. This was the case with Ephraim McDowell who studied with John Bell without receipt of an Edinburgh diploma.

One of the main reasons for the popularity of Edinburgh was the fact that a medical degree could be achieved there in just three years. This was much simpler than the option of going to Oxford or Cambridge and taking 14 years to earn what was essentially the same degree. Other important reasons for Edinburgh's popularity included the fact that it was a nonreligious university owned by the city of Edinburgh. Thus classes were available to anyone who could pay, e.g. dissenters, Jews, and Catholics, versus Oxford and Cambridge where students had to be members of the Church of England.

In Edinburgh's later years, the process became even simpler; a degree could be had for a fee with letters that attested to the character of the individual applying for the degree. The most expensive part of an Edinburgh education was the diploma fee. Thus, many students attended Edinburgh but received their degrees from St. Andrews, Aberdeen, or Rheims just by paying a cheap fee. Such schools became diploma factories, giving out degrees to anyone willing to pay, regardless of skill level.

Edinburgh ultimately changed this policy, mostly because physicians who had studied for their degrees complained that giving out diplomas to anyone demeaned the degree. Medical students were required to take courses such as physics, chemistry, materia medica, anatomy, midwifery, and clinical lectures in the infirmary. After two or three years, the student would present a thesis in Latin, with a copy provided to each professor. The student then underwent an examination. The first day, the student was asked questions about illnesses with diagnosis and treatment. Then, the student had to present written commentaries on Hippocrates and had to defend his thesis against two professors. Finally, the student received his medical degree. Some American students who went abroad to obtain their medical education prior to the Revolutionary war included Thomas Bulfinch, Sylvester Gardiner, Lloyd Zachary, Thomas Cadwallader, Thomas and Phineas Bond, John Redman, Hall Jackson, James Lloyd, John Jones, William Shippen Jr., John Morgan, Adam Kuhn, Samuel Bard, and Benjamin Rush (Table 2.2).

Most medical students in the colonies did not have the option or financial resources to attend a medical school such as Oxford or Edinburgh. Instead, they were trained under the apprenticeship system. The apprenticeship period could last anywhere from one to seven years, with the average time being about three years. The aspiring doctor's father would contract the local medical practitioner for his son to learn "the art and mystery of his craft" (Reiss).

The beginning apprentice would usually be 14 to 16 years old. He was required to do odd jobs around the medical office such as sweeping floors, running errands, and even doubling as the doctor's butler when the doctor had social functions at the house. The apprentice would generally take care of the horses and carriage as well as mix the physician's pills, powders, and concoctions. In his spare time he might do some reading from the physician's library, which usually consisted of only a few books. The apprentice would follow the practitioner on his rounds, and in between visits to houses they would discuss the next case. If the apprentice's family was wealthy enough, they might pay the doctor with money. Dr. Thomas Bond of Philadelphia received 100 pounds from his apprentice for lessons. Quite often, a physician might take on more than one apprentice. The notable Dr. Benjamin Rush had seven apprentices. The apprentice on many occasions married the doctor's daughter as well.

The physician was required not only to teach the student, but also to provide the general upkeep and well being of the apprentice. He had to provide the student with bed, board, and clothing to wear. Teaching consisted mainly of observation and, later on, hands-on training. The apprentice depended on his observation and memory.

When the apprenticeship was over, his master would decide whether he was competent to receive the title of "doctor." The master might give the apprentice a test, or base his opinion on observing the apprentice at work. Diplomas were not issued to qualifying apprentices. The master would give the apprentice a certificate describing the competence of the trainee in the various branches of medicine. This certificate was not a license to practice medicine. It was an acknowledgement that the new doctor was proficient in medicine.

A question debated by medical historians is whether apprentice-trained doctors were as knowledgeable and proficient as the university-trained physicians. University-trained doctors had superior book knowledge, and apprentice-trained doctors had more hands-on experience. The university-trained physician would have been better versed in the subtle philosophical distinctions between medical theories but would lack the clinical experience gained by the apprentice-trained physician.

Despite the increasing number of students graduating from European universities, one can assume that the best of these European physicians would have chosen to stay home, in the civilized world, instead of coming into the unknown of a wilderness area. Many American practitioners followed medical practices that were more harmful to their patients than good. These practices were represented to a great degree by Heroic Medicine, in which the patient would be at the center of suffering due to the use of excessive bleeding, purgatives, emetics, and other severe bodily measures, all considered to be heroic in nature. Both university- and apprentice-trained physicians were guilty in this respect. The statements of university-trained physicians about the need for medical schools should be taken with a grain of salt. These men were more likely to believe in the value of a university degree because they themselves possessed one.

Table 2.2. Some of the First American Students Attending European Schools Prior to the Revolutionary War

Student	Origin	Place Attended Abroad
Thomas Bulfinch (1694-1757)	Boston	London (Under Cheselden), Paris
Lloyd Zachary (1701-1756)	Philadelphia	London (Under Cheselden)
Sylvester Gardiner (1707-1786)	Rhode Island, Boston	London (Under Cheselden), Paris
Thomas Cadwallader (1708-1779)	Philadelphia	London (Under Cheselden), Rheims
Thomas Bond (1712-1784)	Maryland, Philadelphia	Paris
Phineas Bond (1717-1775)	Maryland, Philadelphia	Leyden, Paris, Edinburgh, London
John Redman (1722-1807)	Philadelphia	Edinburgh, London, Paris, Leyden
Hall Jackson (1739-1797)	Porstmouth, NH	London (Association with Withering)
James Lloyd (1728-1810)	Long Island, Boston	London (Under Cheselden, Sharpe, William Hunter)
Thomas Bulfich Son (1728-1802)	Boston	London, Edinburgh
John Jones (1729-1791)	Long Island	London (Under Hunter, McKenzie, Pott), Rheims, Paris, Leyden, Edinburgh
William Shippen, Jr. (1736-1808)	Philadelphia	London (Under John and William Hunter, Hewson, McKenzie), Edinburgh
John Morgan (1735-1789)	Philadelphia	London (Under William Hunter), Edinburgh, Paris
Adam Kuhn (1741-1817)	Philadelphia	Upsala (Under Linnaeus), Edinburgh, France, Holland, Germany
Samuel Bard (1742-1821)	Philadelphia, New York	London, Edinburgh
Benjamin Rush (1745-1813)	Philadelphia	Edinburgh, London, France

Educated European Physicians Migrating to the Colonies

Some educated physicians, mainly from England and Scotland, migrated to the colonies during the colonial period. In this group, we find names such as Charles Chauncey (1592-1672), minister-physician who obtained his MD at Cambridge and became the second president of Harvard College; Thomas Boylston (father of Zabdiel) who secured his MD from Oxford and practiced near Boston, Massachusetts; John Mitchell (d. 1768), who earned an MD in England and settled in Virginia; and Giles Firmin (1615-1697), an "independent apothecary physician, sometime servant of Dr. Clerk of London" (Gordon) who practiced medicine in the English colonies. Of the early physicians, the first one was Lambert Wilson, who began his lectures years before Firmin. Thomas Thatcher (1620-1678), physician and minister who arrived from England in 1635, wrote the first article published in the English colonies. He was a learned man, a scholar in many areas including Arabic, Hebrew, Logic, and Mechanics.

Cadwallader Colden (1688-1776) graduated from Edinburgh and came to Philadelphia in 1710, Gustavus Brown (1689-1765) came from Dalkeith, Scotland, to Maryland in 1708 as a surgeon's mate. Lionel Chalmers graduated from Edinburgh and settled in South Carolina; Peter Middleton (d. 1781) came from Scotland to New York around 1750 and was one of the founders of King's College Medical School in 1768. Alexander Garden (1728-1792) graduated from Edinburgh and settled in Charleston, South Carolina, where he practiced medicine for about thirty years. James Craik (1731-1814) graduated from Edinburgh and settled in Virginia. Alexander Baron and William Brown, were also among the many medical practitioners coming from Scotland.

Samuel Clossey graduated from Dublin University and settled in New York where he was the first Professor of Anatomy in King's Medical School. William MacNeven (1763-1841) from Ireland, graduated from the University of Vienna in 1783 and came to the United States in 1805, where he had several positions in the faculty of King's College Medical School and thereafter in Rutgers Medical College.

Laws Regulating Physicians in the Colonies

The first eighteenth century law definitely benefited the university-trained physician. This law, enacted by the Virginia legislature in 1736, was more concerned with protecting patients than improving medical care. This law specified charges for medical services such as standard fees for town visits and fees based on mileage for out-of-town medical visits. This law also gave university-trained physicians the legal right to charge twice the fees that apprentice-trained doctors were allowed to charge. To provide patients with protection against unsafe drugs, the law required physicians to specify the drugs that were put on the patient's bill. One could say that this was the first "truth-in-advertising" law. This law was allowed to lapse at the end of two years. After the two years, several other bills were introduced to the Virginia legislature, but none passed.

New York adopted its first medical law in 1739. This ordinance required every midwife to swear an oath before the mayor recorder and alderman, on pain of a fine of forty shillings if she did not. This law was more concerned with the ethical conduct of midwives than their medical qualifications. For example, the law stated: "You shall swear, first you shall be Diligent and Faithful and ready to help every woman labouring of child as well the poor as the rich; and in that time of necessity you shall not forsake or leave the poor woman to go to the rich" (Beck). The law even mentioned that midwives had a duty not to conceal the birth of bastard children and had to report to the city alderman the knowledge of the birth. New York also attempted to regulate physicians in 1760. The regulation stated:

> No persons whatsoever should practice as a physician or a surgeon, in the city of New York, before he shall have been examined by one of his majesty's council, the judges of the supreme court, the kings attorney general, and the mayor of the city of New York, for the time being; or by any 3 or more of them, taking this assignment for such exam such proper person or persons as they in their discretion shall think of it (Beck).

The fine for non-compliance of this sort was £5. This was enacted to try to regulate the practice of medicine, which up to this point had few restrictions. It was an attempt to increase the quality of the practitioner. Unfortunately, little effort was made to enforce the law. No record appears of anyone convicted for practicing medicine without a license.

In 1772, the New Jersey Medical Society also tried to enact a medical licensure law, quite similar to the earlier New York law. As in New York, this law was not enforced. Only two more attempts were made to put some type of medical regulation into law. Both attempts failed. No really effective laws were made until after the American Revolution. While ineffective, these attempts highlight the community's recognition that some physicians were of questionable competency.

Table 2.3. Pre-Civil War Local Medical Societies Designated as State Medical Societies		
Date of Founding	Name of Society	Membership Composition
1766	Medical Society of New Jersey	Most of the early members lived in Essex and Middlesex Counties
1781	Massachusetts Medical Society	Society activities and many members in Boston
1789	Medical Society of South Carolina	Limited to Charleston
1791	Medical Society of the State of New York	Limited to New York City
1804	Medical Society of Georgia	Limited to Savannah
1821	Medical Society of Virginia	Most members lived in Richmond
1830	Medical Society of Tennessee	Most members lived in Nashville area
1837	Medical Society of Missouri	Limited to St. Louis, and reorganized as St. Louis Medical Society in 1850
1847	Alabama Medical Society	Limited to Selma, and name changed to Selma Medical Society in 1867

From Rothstein, *American Physicians in the Nineteenth Century: From Sects to Science*.

Fees caused the biggest rift between patients and physicians. The law was asked to intervene or settle disputes on a regular basis. Sometimes fees were paid on a yearly basis for as much or as little as the family would use his services. Payments were made with either money or in such goods as tobacco or corn. The annual fees varied but were usually £5 for apprenticed physicians and £10 for university-educated physicians. This was far too expensive for most colonists, so the use of irregulars such as midwives, quacks, barber-surgeons, apothecaries, and cleric-physicians continued to rise. This popularity of irregulars was one of the physicians' reasons to seek medical regulation. Physicians started to consider the formation of societies to obtain recognition of their functions and rights. In 1766, the first medical society was established in New Jersey. Such societies would continue to develop (Table 2.3).

Different Types of Medical Practitioners of the Colonies

Medicine Men

One of the most important practitioners of the day was the traditional Indian medicine man. The knowledge they bore and the treatments they used were not so different from that of the Europeans, but their plants and herbs made their contributions great. They developed about 170 preparations that are in or have been in the United States pharmacopoeia or National Formulary. Over 50 species of plants in the current British Herbal Pharmacopoeia originated in North America. Native Americans used many preparations that worked, but many did not. They used them based upon trial and error and observation. One drawback to these new remedies was that quacks would go around to carnivals and put on shows to draw people's attention. The quacks would then try to sell their "Indian cures" to the unsuspecting, often using Indian names for their concoctions. After using whatever means they could to sell their medicines, they would leave town.

Surgeons and barber-surgeons

The barber-surgeon's work was considered a craft and was regulated by guild rules. To train potential surgeons, an apprenticeship of seven years was required. The apprentice learned mostly by observation. Theoretically, barber-surgeons could not practice medicine, but they frequently found themselves acting as general practitioners. Barbers and surgeons were both authorized to perform surgery. Barbers did not just cut hair; they also treated the sick. Barbers could shave, cut hair, and draw teeth. Primarily, surgeons did bloodletting. But, they also performed amputations, removed tumors, set fractures, treated lameness, dressed ulcers, pulled teeth, and excised cancers. They also performed lithotomies, the surgical removal of bladder stones.

Bladder stones were a very serious problem for people in the colonial era. The pain they generated was so intense that many people were willing to subject themselves to life-threatening, painful surgeries. There was no means of proper anesthesia, so the patient felt every cut that the surgeon made. This particular surgery had a 50% mortality rate. One method used by surgeons to remove stones was for the surgeon to put his left index finger in the patient's rectum. He then pressed his right hand on the suprapubic area to push the stone down until it bulged into the perineum. He quickly made a transverse incision in front of the anus and through the bladder at the trigone and then pushed out the stone by the finger in the rectum. If a surgeon was competent, he might complete this surgery in under two minutes.

For many of their therapies, surgeons also performed bleeding. The basilic vein of the arm was considered the safest and easiest site to use, but other sites might be used, depending on the problem of the patient. For example, the jugular vein was opened in inflammation of the throat, eye disorders, and affections of the head. Both jugular veins would be compressed to distend the one that was to be opened. A surgeon might also bleed from the tongue, external hemorrhoidal veins, and even the penis. He even used bleeding to treat fractures. The patient would be bled to faintness to relax the muscles, and the bone was put back into place.

To treat a wound, the surgeon might use a tourniquet. If a tourniquet could not be used, the surgeon would use pieces of cloth dipped in copper sulfate instead. If the wound was deep, it was filled with soft lint and covered with cloth dipped in oil. This was kept in place with a roller bandage and not touched for two days. If the patient developed inflammation around the wound, a poultice of bread, milk, butter, and sweet oil was applied. If the patient had not lost too much blood from the wound, he was treated with further bleeding. The effectiveness of such treatments was questionable at a minimum.

Apothecaries

Another type of medical practitioner was the apothecary, also trained by apprenticeship similar to the apprenticeship of a physician. The apprenticeship of an apothecary might last from four to seven years. The student would learn his trade mostly through observation and hands-on training. Since many physicians would refuse to "dirty their hands" in the making of medicines, the patient would have to take a physician's prescription to the local apothecary.

Apothecaries could also act as physicians. However, their range of diagnosis was very limited. All that was involved was asking few questions, looking at the patient, and feeling the pulse. Physicians also made diagnoses by such circumscribed methods. After making a diagnosis, the apothecary would mix the right prescription to treat the disease. The prescription of drugs was imprecise. Colonists had to rely on English ships to send them drugs. Sometimes supply ships would not arrive in time, and other remedies had to be used. The main substitutes were indigenous plants. Neither apothecaries nor physicians had the benefit of standard drug lists or pharmacopoeias.

Many people mistrusted physicians and sought an apothecary for treatment. Apothecaries' methods were less aggressive and therefore less harmful than those of physicians. They charged less money as well.

Midwives

Midwives were always women and rarely had any training or instruction in medicine. This distinguished profession began in remote antiquity when females were required to help each other in times of childbirth. In colonial times, the midwife dealt with the birthing process. A physician would only be called in the case of a very difficult birth. This was true until the middle of the 1700's when Dr. James Lloyd and Dr. William Shippen, Jr. entered obstetrics. It was said that these two men "...deserve especial commendation; as having led the way in overcoming deep-rooted prejudices and in transferring to the profession, from the hands of ignorant and uneducated females, the practice of a different art" (Beck). This did not, however, diminish the use of midwives. When the first medical colleges were formed in the United States, they offered courses in midwifery.

The healthiest communities saw one in every ten children die before their fifth birthday. In more sickly communities this rate would increase to three in ten. Frequent childbearing and poor obstetric practices accounted for much of the mortality among women of the colonial period. In colonial America, women gave birth at home, usually assisted by female family members, neighbors, and a midwife if available. Skilled midwives were highly valued, and in many communities they were given a salary or a house rent-free. Despite their best intentions and skill, they were not respected by physicians. Between 1 and 1.5 percent of all births ended in the mother's death, and her lifetime chance of dying in childbirth was 1 in 8. Many women feared childbirth and had a feeling of impending death.

Midwives were mostly older women, who had children. Having had their own children, they were experienced in the process of childbirth and knew what to expect. It was often said that midwives had experience, and physicians had knowledge. This was why women were more apt to rely on the services of a midwife than those of a physician. Midwives could deliver many babies in their time of service. Elizabeth Phillips of New England is said to have delivered some 3,000 babies, and Lydia Robinson reportedly delivered 1,200 babies in a 35 year period without losing a single mother or baby.

Midwives used mainly herbal remedies. To relieve the discomfort of delivery, midwives might use herbs gathered previously from fields and gardens. Even the husband would be involved in the process of gathering herbs. "Nicholas Gilman went into the woods to gather betony, which was crushed, clarified the juice, and then made it into a syrup with double its weight of sugar. This was then used when his wife went into labor four months later" (Ulrich). Fresh butter was used to lubricate the midwife's hands and to anoint the vagina and perineum to facilitate stretching during labor.

Midwives did more than help with childbirth; they were an integral part of the medical community. Midwives treated illnesses such as snake bites, broken bones, upset stomachs, and burns. Martha Ballard, a midwife made famous by Laurel Thatcher Ulrich, had quite a diverse practice. In addition to midwifery, she helped out during the scarlet fever epidemic. On June 16, Martha Ballard wrote, I "find his wife & child very ill. tarried all night, watch Thomas Sewalls children have the rash, Becky very poorly" (Martha Ballard's Diary Online). Ballard spent a good deal of time treating many patients during this epidemic.

Ballard's job as midwife extended beyond medicine. As a midwife, she was required to take the testimony of an out-of-wedlock mother at birth. During the actual birth, the midwife would ask the mother who the father was. It was thought that during the birthing process, women were unable to lie, so this was seen as the best time to question them. Ballard, like other midwives, would have to question these women and report to the town magistrate the name of the child's father.

Clerics

Clerics were another group of irregulars drawn into service because they were cheap or free, had some level of education, and were trusted. They merely dabbled in medicine and did the best job they could. Another reason for their use was to try to cleanse the soul through spirituality since many believed that disease was God's punishment. The minister was, therefore, a logical choice to address a medical problem. The minister-physician thrived in Puritan New England and the Anglican colonies. Ministers began to choose medicine as a back-up profession for them if the ministry fell through. This was particularly true in England when the Stuart kings were attempting to move the Anglican church towards Catholicism, and many ministers feared being dismissed from the practice of ministry.

Ministers

Ministers were theoretically well prepared to fill the functions of a doctor. They were often the best-educated individuals in their community. Also, they were well informed of medical events that went on in their communities such as births, diseases, accidents, and deaths. Most ministers had access to at least one or two medical books that they could rely on to help treat their patients. A lot of these minister-physicians also kept extensive diaries of medical events, often with various "remarkable providences" and other natural phenomena thought to offer clues to God's will.

Notable Physicians of Mid- and Late Colonial Times

Some distinguished physicians were among the practitioners who migrated to English colonial America. Virginia had the initial medical settlers arrive to Jamestown in 1607. Massachusetts continued with a series of important health care practitioners beginning with the early settlement of Plymouth in 1620 and advancing through the next two centuries (Table 2.4). The other colonies also contributed to the enhancement of medical practice in the developing continent. The colony of Pennsylvania had a large number of physicians who had attended British universities (Table 2.2). A number of distinguished English doctors known for their ability to teach migrated to Pennsylvania. John Kearsley, Sr. (1685-1772) came from England to Philadelphia in 1711 and developed a large practice. He had multiple American apprentices such as Thomas Cadwallader, William Shippen Jr., Lloyd Zachary, John Redman, and Samuel Bard. John Redman in his own right had two distinguished students, William Shippen Jr. and Benjamin Rush. The colony of New York also benefited from a group of notable physicians from Europe and America that influenced the medical practice of the times. Other physicians of repute during colonial times have been described throughout this report.

Probably the most influential minister-physician of the high colonial period was Cotton Mather (1663-1728), the son of Increase Mather, a very prominent minister of the time. Mather received his education from Harvard College, where he acquired his BA in 1678 and his MA in 1681. He was a deeply spiritual man who was well read and wrote on the subjects of religion, science, and history. He tried to heal his parishioners' spiritual and physical ailments. Mather believed that the body was a "divine piece of mechanism," and felt that the humoral theory was valid in that the stomach was the body's "main wheel." He vaguely believed in an animalcular hypotheses or germ theory. He also believed in witchcraft which would later earn him notoriety during and after the Salem witch trials. He married three times and had fifteen children, ten of whom died young to infectious diseases such as smallpox and the measles. He loved his wives and lived much longer than them. He felt that a woman could perform equally in the healing arts and defended their ability. Mather taught his daughter to heal although women practicing in this arena were not always accepted.

Mather himself was self-educated in the field of medicine, having been an avid reader of medical literature. In addition to practicing medicine, Mather wrote medical works. His most famous medical book was *The Angel of Bethesda*. He began this work in the 1720s, but the book was not actually published until the twentieth century. It is now recognized as one of the great books of its time. In it, Mather provides a clear description of what would become the germ theory, suggesting the specificity of animalculae and their means of transmission, even pointing out that healthy bodies could often resist invasion. An avid reader of medical theory, Mather obtained this idea from the work of Athanasius Kircher (1602-1680), whose work with the microscope led him to theorize that the tiny animals he had seen with the microscope were the cause of disease. Mather took the theory a step further. He believed that these tiny animals were the cause of smallpox.

In 1713, Mather was elected a Fellow of the Royal Society of London for his scholarly work. This gave him not only prestige but access to the society's literature. It is there he found manuscripts describing smallpox inoculation as practiced in Turkey. He also learned of smallpox inoculation from his African slave Onesimus, who told him of African ways to prevent smallpox. This began his commitment to bringing inoculation to the forefront of American society.

In 1721, the British warship *H.M.S. Seahorse* from Barbados docked in Boston harbor, carrying smallpox. By autumn, the disease had spread throughout Boston, Cambridge, and Charlestown, with death rates hitting 50%. Mather tried to find a way to save his family from the dreaded disease. He recalled what he had learned of inoculation and preached from his pulpit, trying to get other doctors of the area to accept the practice. Only Zabdiel Boylston (1679-1766) took up the challenge.

Table 2.4. Some Other Physicians of Repute in Virginia and Massachusetts during Colonial Times

Virginia	Massachusetts
William Gulstone (b. & d. unkown)	Samuel Fuller (1580-1633)
John Mitchell (d. 1768)	Giles Firmin (1615-1697)
John Clayton (1693-1773)	Thomas Thatcher (1620-1678)
William Cabell (1700-1774)	Zabdiel Boylston (1679-1766)
Thomas Walker (1715-1794)	Nathaniel Williams (1675-1783)
James Craik (1731-1814)	Benjamin Doolittle (1695-1738)
Elisha Cullen Dick (1762-1825)	Simon Tufts (1700-1747)
James McClurg (1745-1823)	Sylvester Gardiner (1707-1786)
William Baynham (1749-1814)	Ezekiel Hersey (1709-1770)
	Edward Holyoke (1728-1829)
	Josiah Bartlett (1729-1795)
	Oliver Prescott (1731-1804)
	Cotton Tuffs (1731-1815)
	Samuel Danforth (1740-1827)
	Joseph Warren (1741-1775)
	William Aspinwall (1743-1823)
	William Baylies (1743-1826)
	John Jefferies (1745-1819)
	John Warren (1753-1815)

Boylston was a family friend of Mather and a well-known surgeon and physician who had learned medicine by apprenticeship. He trained under Dr. John Cutter of Boston. A native of Brookline, Massachusetts, Boylston was the first colonial-born surgeon. He once cut off a woman's breast, curing her of what would later be termed cancer, after doctors had tried to cure her for years. He also removed several gallstones in his practice. He later became the first born American to be celebrated in England. He later lectured at the Royal College of Physicians and was received with exceptional honor at the Royal Society.

Introduction of Inoculation to the English Colonies

The inoculation method suggested by Mather and put into practice by Boylston remains as a clear example of a very successful practical experiment. But not everyone agreed with the idea. Mather's biggest opponent was Dr. William Douglass (1691-1752). Douglass, a Scottish physician who immigrated to New England in 1716, was the only MD in Boston in 1721 and had become quite influential. He was backed by the medical profession and the newspapers. He was the most voluminous writer in the colonial period but was a bitter person. Douglass wrote in a work published posthumously in 1753 that "in general, the physical practice in our colonies is so perniciously bad, that excepting in surgery, and some very acute cases, it is better to let nature, under a proper regimen, take her course, then to trust to the honesty and sagacity of the practitioner" (Beck). Douglass also wrote about the colonial physician "Frequently there is more danger from the physician, than from distemper… but sometimes not withstanding the male practice, nature gets the better of the doctor and the patient recovers" (Beck). He vehemently opposed variolation (a form of smallpox inoculation) and was very critical of uneducated practitioners and clerics who meddled in medicine. This perhaps explains some of his disdain for Boylston and Mather. Douglass claimed that Boylston was a uncertified quack and stated that Mather and Boylston were medical dilettantes, using their standing to foist risky inoculations on an unwilling public.

Smallpox was a dreaded disease, unrivaled in its detrimental effects. It was the most feared disease of the colonial period. It was highly contagious, spread by inhalation and contact with sores, victims' clothing, or contaminated bedding. Typical treatment is described by Rev. Thomas Thatcher: "let the sick abstain from flesh and wine, and open air, let him use small beer warmed with a toast for his ordinary drink, and moderately when desires it." The sick ate gruel, potage, boiled apples, and milk. No real understanding of the disease process was evident in the colonies.

Inoculation was the single most important practical therapeutic development in colonial America. Mather speculated that smallpox might be an animalculated disease, and that finding was later confirmed by viewing the pustules left by the smallpox under a microscope. After reading articles about Turkish inoculations and talking to African slaves regarding inoculation practices, Mather suggested inoculating all the peoples of the American colonies to rid the land of smallpox for good. Some of Mather's children had died from smallpox, and he wanted to find a way to stop the spread of the disease and protect others. After approaching several of the New England physicians, Mather turned to Boylston, and the two set out to inoculate others. Boylston performed the inoculations, and Mather pushed for them.

On June 26, 1721, Boylston inoculated his six-year-old son and two of his slaves. All took on mild cases of smallpox and then recovered. They all showed resistance to further exposures. The inoculations were done by collecting fresh pus from smallpox victims' sores, putting a drop on a sharp knife and cutting the skin of a healthy person. This would be mixed with the blood of the healthy person and covered with a bandage, thus inducing a mild case of the pox. By July 10 of that year, ten people had been inoculated. By early 1722, Boylston had performed 247 inoculations, while two other physicians had performed 39 more. Of that number, only six had died; the rest were immune. Two months earlier in England, inoculations began to appear there. Neither country knew of the other's efforts at first, and when the results came out, each country's inoculators cited the other's work.

Douglass's supporters were clearly annoyed and accused Mather of being insanely irresponsible. Douglass himself was furious, suggesting that Mather and Boylston were trying to intervene in the punishment set forth by God and that giving these people pox was not only immoral but extremely dangerous. James Franklin, publisher of the *New England Courant* and more famous as the older brother of Benjamin Franklin, included many essays against inoculation in his paper. Puritan ministers rose up in favor of what Boylston was doing, but the papers and medical professionals were up in arms. Ironically, the ministers were in favor of inoculating against a disease supposedly caused by a judging God upon his flock, while the physicians, who would rather look to the side of science for some answers, were against it. The Boston Newsletter called Boylston an uncertified quack, so illiterate he couldn't have read the Society articles that Mather had given him. Boston outlawed inoculations and ordered all who had been inoculated and those who were seeking inoculation to Spectacle Island Hospital. The inoculations continued in spite of this plea. Douglas wanted Mather and Boylston tried for attempted murder. In November 1721, someone tossed a lit bomb into Mather's study window at three o'clock in the morning. Fortunately, it hit a chair inside Mather's house which caused the fuse to fall out. Attached to the bomb was a note that read, "Cotton Mather, you dog, Dam you: I'll inoculate you with this, with a pox to you." Boylston was forced to hide for two weeks so that a lynch mob could not find him. Many applauded the attackers but law enforcement put a £50 reward to help find the assailants. Meanwhile the inoculations continued.

No one had died from receiving the inoculation by the end of 1721, but that did not squelch the threats against the two. Boylston and Mather said that their results showed that only one inoculee had died from the inoculations and that she had likely contracted the disease before being inoculated. They said that only a small number of poxes erupt on the skin with their procedure thereby relieving the "pox marks" on victims faces. This was not always true, and in fact numerous, sometimes even hundreds of eruptions did occur. The inoculees were allowed to have visitors and wander around with open sores that could then infect others with the more potent traditional way of getting smallpox. It was felt at first that inoculation prevented one from passing the disease via the traditional route. This was not so, and those revelations added fuel to the already hot flames against inoculations. Skeptics were noting how reckless the two were being and charged that they were endangering the public's safety.

Boylston and Mather's evidence encouraged certain English physicians in their support of inoculation. For more than twenty years many fought against the practice, but the evidence was overwhelming. The results were evident. Of the 286 persons inoculated only six had died, a one to two percent mortality rate. Of those not inoculated, in the 1721-1722 outbreak, there were 5,579 cases resulting in 844 deaths. That's a mortality rate of 15 percent. Eventually the tide would turn, and inoculation would become an accepted practice. For some time, instead of giving them thanks and accolades, Boylston and Mather received rage and scorn. Benjamin Franklin, after seeing the evidence, reversed his disdain for the practice and became a vocal leader for the use of inoculations. It was not until the American Revolution over a half century later that the practice became widespread; George Washington showed his belief in inoculations when he had the entire Continental Army inoculated during the Revolutionary War. It is worthy to note, however, that had there not been skeptics, mass inoculations would have occurred without safety measures in place such as isolating the inoculee until the sores were gone. The skeptics did have their place in history but if it weren't for the steadfast faith of Mather and Boylston, thousands of people would have died unnecessarily. Two years after the epidemic, Dr. Boylston was invited to London to lecture at the Royal College of Physicians and received an honorary membership in the Royal Society of London. There is also speculation that he inoculated the royal family upon his visit and that his wealth upon retiring was due to a grateful crown.

Other Diseases Besides Smallpox

Although the fight against smallpox was a dominant theme in the colonial period, it was by no means the only disease present. Many "remedies," all of them ineffectual, existed. Disease was rampant in this new land.

Many diseases, including hookworm, dengue fever, and yellow fever, were of African descent. Seaports were always threatened with new outbreaks of all kinds of diseases as the arrival of each ship brought more infected persons into the new colonies. There was relatively good health in colonial settlements for the first few years because towns were small and visitors rare. As the cities got bigger, sanitary conditions went from poor to disastrous, and water supplies were contaminated. Some early diseases, including typhoid, dysentery, and malaria, were common due to this infected water supply. Infected mosquitoes became more prevalent and, as such, created large breeding grounds for disease. Body lice also led to typhus fever. In Massachusetts, the city of Charlestown moved their entire town across the river to what is now Boston because the city had become so contaminated that the settlers had no choice. Scurvy was still present because many people could not get citrus fruits.

Most people tried to treat themselves first and resorted to a doctor only when their own treatments were ineffective. In rural areas, home remedies and self-medication meant life or death to people who were far away from a doctor. The mother, in her role as caregiver, was a natural choice for the family doctor. She often brought medical recipes from her own mother that could be used. As the cook of the family, she knew that energy and health depended on good food. In times of illness, she would have a store of recipes that were used. She had quite a few recipes for easy to digest foods such as whey, barley water, toast, apple water, soups, gruel, porridges, and calf's feet jelly. Many illnesses such as insect bites, burns, poison ivy, coughs and colds, bruises and sprains needed to be treated. Colonists would make up simple lotions, syrups, and salves to treat these injuries. Most of their treatments methods used indigenous plants. For example, Martha Ballard used many local plants to treat her patients such as tansy, tow, turnips, wormwood, yarrow, and honey.

Disease trends are hard to track because there is little statistical data from the time, and what is present is hard to discern because they did not classify diseases in the same way that we classify them now. Each settler brought his own diseases to the new land, including many diseases brought by African immigrants. The Native Americans were a healthy race, and this New World had few widespread diseases before these immigrants' arrival. These new diseases decimated the Native Americans and are the reason for the widespread death and collapse of their society. The new arrivals were broken down with scurvy from the lack of fresh citrus fruits on their long journey here. This made them more susceptible to other diseases, and the medical community was ill prepared for the tasks set before them.

Medical Books and Other Publications

The only medical books available in the colonies were books brought over from England. Only two medical publications appeared in the colonies before 1696. These included Thomas Thatcher's *A Brief Rule to Guide the Common-People of New England How to Order Themselves and Theirs in the Small Pocks, or Measles* (1678) and John Oliver's *A Present To Be Given to Teeming Women* (1694). Another publication was written by Thomas Palmer (1666-1743). His work, *Admirable Secrets of Physick and Chyrugery*, is a good example of a publication in the Americas that was specifically for the use of the colonists. In this, Palmer lists many diseases, and the best way to treat them. He mentions how to cure a headache by opening a vein in the forehead. He also puts forth how to cure smallpox, "the cure of this is to open a vein before the 4th day and before spots appear. If the body be bound at the beginning, a gentle purge of syrup of roses and sienna or cassias is good." Palmer also describes how to treat madness. He advises the use of frequent bleeding in the left arm, and the use of leeches. Vomits should be used, along with the boiled brains of a dog. All these remedies were collected by Palmer from midwives and doctors for the use of common, everyday people.

Colonists also would use information from almanacs and medical literature from England to guide them in their treatments. Some of the more popular publications in the colonies were *English Physician* (1652), *Every Man His Own Doctor* (1734), and *Domestic Medicine* (1769). Benjamin Franklin also published *Poor Richard's Almanack*, which had articles on such things as dissolving kidney stones with lemon juice, recipes for gout, cures for worms, and even remedies for pimples.

Another type of publication that summarized the treatments available in the English colonies was a pharmacopoeia. In 1778, a thirty-two page publication by William Brown was the first pharmacopoeia published in English America. This work offered a list of the most available drugs in the English colonies.

Other Medical Treatments

Medical science was not advanced in either its treatments or its reasoning. It was trial by error treatments, and for those that did work, it was due more to luck than skill. There was little reasoning about why things worked or didn't work. There was a feeling that the doctor needed to do something rather than nothing at all. This attitude led to gross overtreatment, especially where bloodletting was concerned. The medicines that did work were generally given in inordinate quantities. Excess was a way of thinking.

For many medical ailments, therapeutic bleeding, or bloodletting, was the recommended treatment. Physicians would drain the body of blood in the belief that the excess blood was causing inflammation and that letting it out would remedy the situation. Bloodletting was used quite frequently in treating fevers. The worse the condition, the more a patient was bled. In some instances, such as severe tonsil edema, the veins under the tongue would be cut. Veins in the "neck holes" were used for some fevers, and the veins on the outside of the ankles were said to relieve hemorrhoids and sciatica. William Cobbett, on the other hand, termed bleeding as "One of the great discoveries which are made, from time to time, for the depopulation of the earth." As brutal as this treatment was, it would become more prevalent under the influence of Benjamin Rush, the great bloodletter. There were many other diseases and treatments of the times. Some were fairly benign while others were more harmful such as the preventive treatment for rickets of dipping a child in cold water every morning until the age of eight or nine.

In the seventeenth century, Peruvian bark (developed into quinine in the 1820s), as previously mentioned, was found to be effective in the treatment of malaria. St. John's wort was used to treat "madness," and is still used today as an over-the-counter anti-depressant. The colonial Pharmacopoeia included St. John's wart, cloeurs, spurge, fennel, saffron, parsley, elder, snake root, roasted rhubarb, and some forms of opiates. Calomel (mercurious chloride) was used to sooth and moisten the throat, a treatment which did have some success. Most plants produced in the colonies such as tobacco and sarsaparilla proved ineffectual for medical purposes but had other uses. The more valuable drugs such as coca, curare, and cinchona bark were native to the Americas. Overall, the treatments were many, the results few.

Hospital Development in the American Colonies

Physicians had virtually no hospitals in which to work. There were some early hospitals with little capability, but they didn't last and had no effect on the medical establishment. The first permanent general hospital in the America was not established until near the end of the colonial period in 1752 at Philadelphia (Figure 1). Dr. Thomas Bond, with the help of Benjamin Franklin, was a significant influence in the construction of the Pennsylvania hospital. He wanted to build a hospital that would have all of the advantages of European hospitals. The colony gave £2000 to start the project with the final £2000 to be raised through public donations. The money was raised quickly, and in 1752 the first patients were admitted into the hospital which was set up in a temporary building until the permanent hospital was built in 1755. Although this was the dawn of modern hospitals, medicine was still practiced by a great number of uneducated physicians. Some medical practitioners viewed illness as a misfortune to be met with and as a punishment for sins.

In 1773, The New York Hospital was established. Because of a damaging fire, the hospital was closed and reopened in 1791. The Massachusetts General Hospital was founded in 1811 but did not open until 1821. Hospitals continued to progress in the now independent United States, and in 1873, there were 178 hospitals with fewer than 50,000 beds. The efficiency of these institutions grew as well. However, hospitals in modern times would become very complex organizations, requiring considerable attention to run them appropriately.

Conclusion

The end of the colonial period saw an improvement in medicine inasmuch as it brought with it more educated physicians. Some European university-trained doctors began to practice in colonial America as stability and opportunity began to take hold in the new land. Minister-physicians such as Cotton Mather contributed a great deal to colonial medicine. Self-educated and apprentice-trained physicians such as Zabdiel Boylston introduced the practice of smallpox inoculation (as suggested by Mather) with extraordinary positive results. This practice was the single most important event in American colonial medicine. Some educated European physicians, who included William Douglass, Cadwallader Colden, Alexander Garden, John Kearsley, and many more, made their mark in American medical life. Important American contributors in late colonial times were represented by John Redman, John Morgan, William Shippen, Jr., Thomas Bond, Casper Wistar, and latecomers such as Benjamin Rush. The American colonies would take great strides forward in the next era as English America's first medical school opened in 1765.

CHAPTER 3
EUROPEANS KNEW MEDICINE BEFORE*

Europe had several esteemed and seasoned universities by the time English Colonial America began its first permanent settlement in 1607. Bologna, Paris, Oxford, and Montpellier were founded in the 1100s; Cambridge, Padua, Salamanca, Toulouse, Siena, and Sevilla in the 1200s; and subsequently, by the 1500s, other new and important universities flourished throughout Europe. Among these institutions were the universities in Avignon in France; Naples, Rome, and Florence in Italy; Valladolid and Huesca in Spain; Vienna in Austria; and Heidelberg and Cologne in Germany. Universities, by definition centers of learning and congregation, housed educational, scientific, medical, and specific related teachings. Medical schools also were spun from recently created universities. Our quest in this chapter is to determine the medical knowledge that Europeans possessed at the time of English colonization.

Table 3.1. Leading Medical Men of Antiquity

Physician	Country of Origin	Teachings
Hippocrates (460-375 BC)	Greece	Rational Approach, Humoral Pathology
Herophilus (c. 300 BC)	Greece	True Nature of Nerves
Erasistratus (c. 260 BC)	Greece	Advanced Study of Causes of Disease
Asclepiades (c. 99 BC)	Greece	Physical Therapeutics
Soranus (c. 90 BC)	Greece	Knowledge of Gynecology
Galen (129-199 AD)	Greece	Humoral Pathology, Surgery

* Partially published in *Southwest Michigan Medical Journal*, 1(1):23-27, 2004, by Toledo-Pereyra LH.

Influence of Medical Men of Antiquity

The medical teachings of the time were predominantly theoretical and were based on the ancient writings of well-known Greek or Greco-Roman master physicians of the likes of Hippocrates (460-377 BC) and Galen (129-199 AD) (Table 3.1). Centuries after Galen's live teachings, his overwhelming influence persisted for centuries. During the Middle Ages, his principles were considered to be unchallengeable. Medical students of the fifteenth and even sixteenth centuries were required to know about the writings of the ancient physicians, to review the medieval writers, and to reason on the nature of disease. They possessed few effective treatments (Table 3.2).

Table 3.2. Noted Physicians of the Middle Ages

Physician	Country of Origin	Teachings
Rhazes (865-925)	Persia	El-Hawi
Avicenna (980-1037)	Persia	Canon of Medicine
Maimonides (1135-1204)	Spain	Aphorisms, Regimen Sanitatis
Gilbertus (1180-1250)	England	Compendium Medicinae
Theodoric (1205-1296)	Italy	Teachings of Surgery
Henri de Mondeville (1260-1320)	France	Surgical Contributions
Guy de Chauliac (1300-1368)	France	Surgical Treatments
John Ardene (1306-1380)	England	Treatise in Surgery

Late Middle Ages and Early Renaissance

In the late Middle Ages and Early Renaissance, practical exercises for teaching medicine were not available in Great Britain, and some British students went mainly to Italian universities, particularly to the University of Padua, for more medical education. That was the case for William Harvey (1578-1657). He received his degree of doctor of physic in 1602 at Padua before returning to Cambridge to receive his doctorate in medicine. In England, William Harvey was so highly regarded that he became the physician to Kings James I and Charles I.

Preceding Harvey, in the mid-Renaissance, two English physicians,

Thomas Linacre (1460-1524), educated in Oxford and founder of the Royal College of Physicians, and John Caius (1510-1573), educated in Cambridge, greatly advanced the knowledge of medicine of the times. Their work in humanism and in the transmission of medical concepts from the Greeks and Romans to English practitioners was well-known. During this period, Andreas Vesalius (1514-1564), a Belgium-trained physician-surgeon, greatly contributed to the characterization of anatomy. Through careful analysis of anatomical structures, he further established the discipline of descriptive and topographical anatomy. In 1543, he published his landmark work, *De Humani Corporis Fabrica,* which would revolutionize the knowledge and understanding of the human body. In a clear and systematic manner, and by using human dissections, he described with extraordinary precision the anatomical elements of the human body. No one before him had reached this pinnacle.

Table 3.3. Distinguished Medical Men of the Renaissance

Medical Scholar	Country of Origin	Contributions
Thomas Linacre (1460-1524)	England	Translation of the Masters
Girolamo Fracastoro (1478-1553)	Italy	Epidemic Diseases
Jacob Sylvius (1478-1555)	France	Anatomical Descriptions
Paracelsus (1493-1541)	Switzerland	Cause and Nature of Disease
Jean Fernel (1497-1558)	France	Physiology and Clinical Medicine
Garcia Da Orta (1501-1568)	Portugal	Compendium on Drugs
Servetus (1509-1553)	Spain	Discovery of Lesser Circulation
Ambroise Pare (1510-1590)	France	Advances in Surgery
John Caius (1510-1573)	England	Enhanced Medicine and Literature
Andreas Vesalius (1514-1564)	Belgium	Founder of Modern Anatomy
Eustachio (1520-1574)	Italy	Anatomical Writings
Fallopio (1523-1562)	Italy	Anatomical Contributions
Fabricius (1537-1619)	Italy	Anatomical Teachings
Tagliacozzi (1545-1599)	Italy	Plastic Surgery Repairs

A few years before Vesalius, Paracelsus (1493-1541) had expressed his disdain for academia and had presented some interesting concepts on the influence of chemistry in disease development and how external causes were at the root of these happenings. Paracelsian medicine was, therefore, based on chemical principles. Paracelsian doctors thought God had enlightened them, and they challenged Galen's theory of medicine, which used botanical remedies. Ambroise Paré (1510-1590), a French surgeon and contemporary of Vesalius, participated in the rise of surgery and put forward important concepts in the management of wounds. He recognized the critical role that anatomy played in medicine and surgery and made contributions to orthopedics and prosthesis development. One of his works, *Method of Treating Wounds* (1545), would be required reading for future surgeons and physicians (Table 3.3).

Late Renaissance and Early Modern Era

William Harvey was the first man to scientifically prove the circulation of the blood. He had studied Galen's theory that the liver makes blood and eventually disproved it through various experiments. He concluded that there was no way the liver could account for the body's entire circulatory volume as proposed in Galen's model. Eventually, he proved that the blood leaves the heart, is pumped through the arteries throughout the body, and later returns to the heart through the veins to make the journey again. To prove his concept, Harvey considered the following possibility:

> If a vein is located, say, in the arm, and pressure is exerted between valves, the venous blood can be seen and felt to flow not back and forth but ineluctably toward the heart. Similarly, if a bandage is wrapped around the arm so as to block the flow of blood through the veins while leaving open arterial flow, the veins (but not the arteries) will swell. If the arteries are also blocked, however, the veins will not swell.

In 1628, Harvey Published *The Movement of the Heart and the Blood (Exercitato Anatomica de Motu Cordis et Sanguineis).* With this book he laid the scientific foundation of experimental medicine and experimental physiology.

University-trained students, then, became learned physicians but with minimal ability to treat the prevalent maladies of the time. Successful therapy for specific diseases had not reached the physician's and patient's world yet. It would take until the development of late modern medicine in the early twentieth century before a clear therapeutic difference would be seen.

When the first permanent English settlers stepped on American soil, most of these enlightening advances had yet to be discovered or widely disseminated. At this point in time, William Harvey, Thomas Sydenham (1624-1689), Marcello Malpighi (1628-1694), Herman Boerhaave (1668-1738), Giovanni Morgagni (1682-1771), and other distinguished physicians had not had the opportunity to make their important and seminal contributions to medical thought and practice (Table 3.4). Even with their contributions, the practice of medicine in English Colonial America was not going to change significantly since these advances did not immediately translate into practical and effective medical diagnosis and treatment. Treatment was not readily forthcoming!

World of Sydenham and Boerhaave

Although Thomas Sydenham was not a professor or teacher of medicine, he "dominated the field of clinical medicine" in the seventeenth century. Sydenham is considered the "English Hippocrates" and the founder of modern clinical medicine. Throughout his lifetime he devoted his studies to the natural history of disease. Sydenham began his studies at Oxford University in 1643 but left after two months because of the English Civil War. In 1647, he returned to Oxford, where he received his bachelors' degree in medicine in 1648. Sydenham did not receive his medical license until 1663 and had been practicing without a license up until that time. He received his doctorate in 1676.

In the 1660s Sydenham was considered the most successful physician of his time. In most cases, he opted for noninvasive treatment such as fresh air and rest. He also opted not to overmedicate his patients. By mixing opium and wine, he would prescribe "Sydenham's laudanum" for pain. He also popularized Peruvian bark in the treatment of malaria and fevers. In 1666, Sydenham published *The Method of Treating Fevers.* Additionally, this physician was responsible for the first accurate description of rheumatism (today known as arthritis). He helped his fellow clinicians immeasurably by separating rheumatism from gout and scarlet fever from measles.

Another luminary of this age was Herman Boerhaave, often called the greatest clinician of modern times. Together with Sydenham, he revived clinical bedside teaching, which originated with Hippocrates. If Sydenham was considered the English Hippocrates, Boerhaave was the European Hippocrates.

Boerhaave had a special recognition and reverence for Sydenham. It was said that every time he spoke his name, he bowed in a sign of consideration for the great English clinician. Although Boerhaave was a great physician, even called the "undisputed master," he did not introduce a diagnostic or therapeutic discovery for which he is known. More importantly, perhaps, he developed a method of clinical diagnosis of special significance today and in those times as well. Boerhaave was able to integrate teaching with observation by taking students to patients' bedsides; this was his simple yet important contribution to medicine. Students flocked from all over the world to attend Boehraave's lectures and to be taught by Boerhaave in the St. Cecilia Hospital at Leyden. In examining corpses for further signs of disease, he gave insights to the clinical method of medical teaching still used today, the clinico-pathological approach to disease. He taught mostly at Leyden.

Boerhaave disagreed with bloodletting, purging, and cauterization; instead he called for careful observation in order to determine the course and causation of the disease. Boerhaave spent a lifetime clarifying and applying physics and chemistry in logical way. He integrated anatomy and pathology into the study of medicine and bedside teaching. By uniting science and observation with patient care, Boerhaave filled a large void in clinical medicine. Herman Boerhaave's publications include *Institutions Medicae*, *Classifications of Disease* (1708), and *The Book of Aphorisms* (1709), which was "a Hippocratic guide to help physicians treat patients." He also wrote *Index Plantarum* (1710), in which he catalogued thousands of plant species and their medicinal properties. Finally, his *Elementa Chemiae*, published in 1732, was the most famous work of his time.

At the age of seventeen, Albrecht von Haller (1708-1777) was attracted to study medicine at Leyden under Boerhaave. He was a most industrious student, receiving his doctorate at the age of nineteen, and he was decidedly Boerhaave's greatest pupil. In terms of individual achievements, he probably stands ahead of his mentor. In the spring of 1736, Haller was appointed professor of medicine, anatomy, and surgical operations at Gottingen, where he remained for seventeen years. As a professor Haller passed on many of the teachings of Boerhaave, and due to his knowledge of the nervous system, he became known as the father of modern irritability and sensibility.

Table 3.4. Distinguished Post-Renaissance Medical Men, of the Early Modern Era, Whose Influence was Evident During the Seventeenth Century

Medical Scholar	Country of Origin	Contribution
Sanctorius (1561-1636)	Italy	Introduced Thermometer and Chronometer
Jean Van Helmont (1577-1644)	Belgium	Chemical Basis of Medicine
William Harvey (1578-1657)	England	Discovery of Great Circulation
Gaspare Aselli (1581-1626)	Italy	Discovery of Lymphatic Circulation
Nicholas Tulp (1593-1674)	Holland	Surgical Contributions
Francis Glisson (1597-1677)	England	Anatomical Discoveries
Athanasius Kircher (1602-1680)	Germany	Microorganisms as Cause of Infectious Diseases
Giovanni Borelli (1608-1679)	Italy	Circulatory Physiology
Nicholas Culpepper (1616-1654)	England	Translated Pharmacopoeia
Daniel Whistler (1619-1684)	England	Description of Clinical Rickets
Thomas Sydenham (1624-1689)	England	Natural History of Disease
Robert Boyle (1627-1691)	England	Chemical Considerations
Marcello Malpighi (1628-1694)	Italy	Capillary Circulation
Anthony van Leeuwenhoek (1623-1723)*	Holland	Microscopic Observations
Hermann Boerhaave (1668-1738)*	Holland	Clinical Medicine
*Their lives continued into the eighteenth century.		

Haller's studies included researches of the mechanics of respiration, the formation of bone, the development of the embryo, and the digestive juices. Most important are his "conceptions of the nature of living substances and of the action of the nervous system" (Sigerist, *The Great Doctors*). In terms of the nervous system, before Haller there was limited knowledge in the understanding of the role of the brain in disease. He was the first to show how the nerves reach the brain, and that those nerves are responsible for sensation. "Haller was a modern physiological thinker" (Sigerist, *The Great Doctors*). He always remained rational, with no mystical or obscure themes.

Haller published several medical books. *Primea Linea Physiologiae* (1747) was considered the "first systematic manual of physiology in medical history." He also published an eight-volume handbook of anatomy and embryology, *Elementa Physiologiae Corpus Humani* (1757-1766).

Influence of the Edinburgh School of Medicine

Alexander Monroe, primus (1697-1767), professor of anatomy and surgery at Edinburgh in 1720, had been a student of Boerhaave at Leyden. His contributions to the medical school added more than any single individual had to its reputation. Progression in the Edinburgh school did not occur until the time of Monroe primus. He was a founder of the Edinburgh Medical School. He taught for nearly forty years and trained his son, Alexander Monroe, secundus (1733-1817). Not only was Alexander Monroe secundus a famous teacher, he was also a great physician. In 1753, Monroe secundus described the interventricular foramen between the lateral ventricles of the brain. When he took over his father's chair, the class consisted of only 190 students. When he handed the chair over to his own son, the class numbered nearly 400 students. Alexander Monroe tertius (1773-1859) was not as prestigious as his father and grandfather. He was rather indifferent to teaching. When he finally resigned his chair in 1846, the three Monroes had held it for over 120 years. John Goodsir (1814-1867) succeeded Monroe tertius in 1864.

William Cullen (1710-1790) was another pillar of the Edinburgh school, where he held the chair of chemistry, materia medica, and the practice of physic. Cullen had graduated from Glasgow and became professor of medicine there in 1751 before going to Edinburgh in 1757. Among Cullen's theories were those on nervous energy. He contended that external stimuli affected the nervous system, which determined nervous energy. Cullen's textbooks were widely used. His *Nosology* was published in 1769, and in 1777 he published *First Lines on the Practice of Physic.* Before American physicians wrote their own manuals of materia medica, Cullen's were considered gospel. He was the teacher of the most distinguished upcoming American physicians of the latter part of the eighteenth century and beginning of the nineteenth century. Included among them were John Redman, John Jones, William Shippen Jr., John Morgan, Adam Kuhn, Benjamin Rush, Thomas Parke, Samuel Griffiths, Phillip Syng Physick, and Caspar Wistar. Most of them would be considered the unmistakable founders of the Medical School of the College of Philadelphia, now known as the University of Pennsylvania Medical School. The influence of Cullen and the Edinburgh school in the medical education of young Americans of the late English colonies was without a doubt unique and of enormous importance.

Influence of John Hunter

John Hunter (1728-1793) was a surgeon, anatomist, physician, and naturalist. He was considered the greatest surgeon of the eighteenth century and is remembered as one of the early founders of modern medicine. He studied under his brother William who was of great repute in London. In May of 1767, Hunter inoculated himself with the purulent material of a man he knew to be infected with gonorrhea. He did this in order to determine if gonorrhea and syphilis were two different diseases, or two different manifestations of the same disease. Little did he know that the man indeed had both gonorrhea and syphilis. And so, he came to the incorrect conclusion that they were manifestations of the same venereal disease, but to his credit Hunter described the chancre of the syphilis so well, that it was named the Hunterian chancre, an honor indeed.

John Hunter—very much like William Cullen—attracted a large number of students from late colonial English America. Able students with economic means would opt for the British Isles, including London and Edinburgh. In the second half of the eighteenth century, the Hunter brothers of London were a required stop for those Americans pursuing credible European training. John Morgan, William Shippen Jr., Caspar Wistar, and Philip Syng Physick were among many of the students who trained under John Hunter. John Hunter exerted a decisive influence in the training of the leading physicians of late colonial English America.

The Hunterian Museum was Hunter's most visible legacy, containing some 13,500 specimens. In collecting for his museum, he was able to see form and function in nature. His museum would also serve as a mold by which all other museums of natural history are modeled. Some of Hunter's publications included his *Treatise on the Blood, Inflammation and Gunshot Wounds*, which was published posthumously in 1794. He also published *Treatise on Venereal Disease* in 1786, and his two-part *Treatise on the Natural History of the Human Teeth* was published in 1771 and 1778.

Table 3.5. Historical Sequence on the Influence of Galen in the Medicine of the English American Colonies

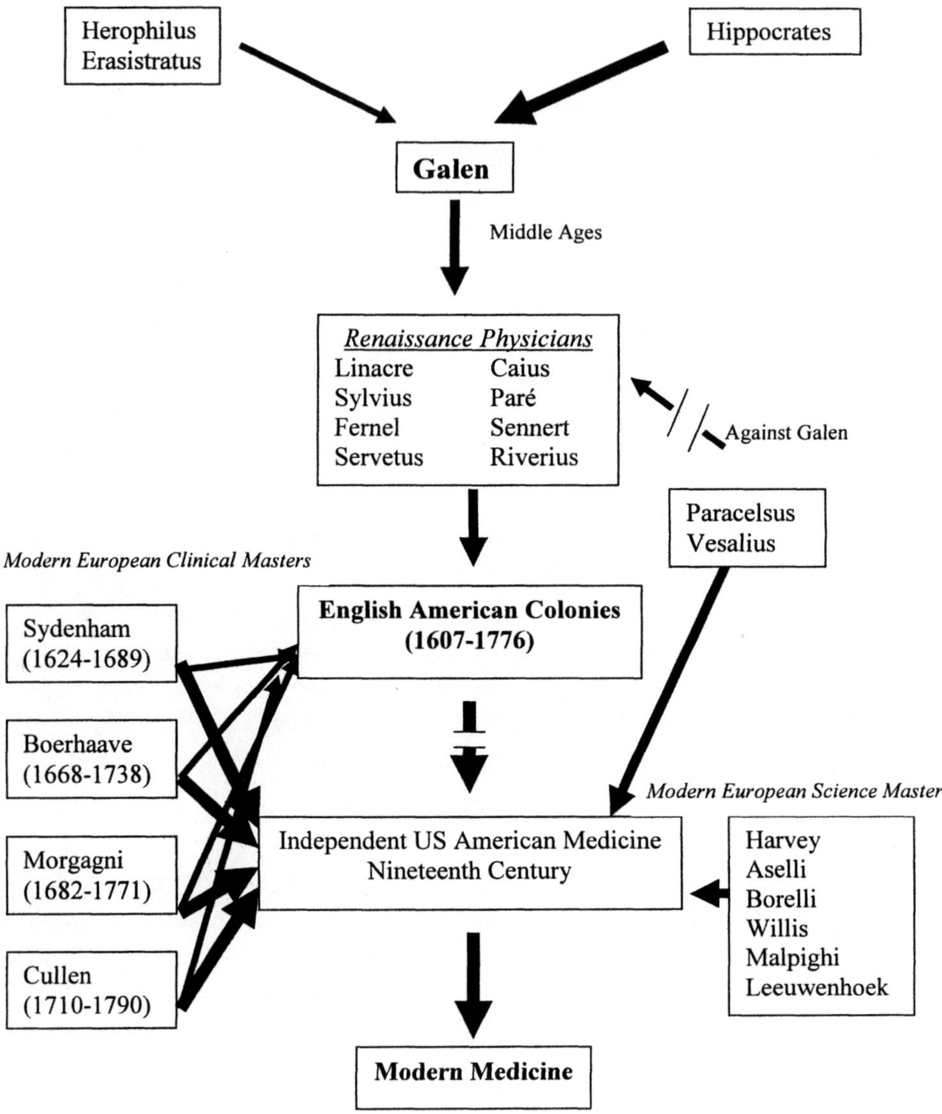

European Physicians Coming to the English American Colonies

The first educated physicians who came to English America arrived centuries before the great majority of European medical teachings had been popularized. Of course, these physicians knew of the works of Hippocrates and Galen, and probably Avicenna. Additionally these physician immigrants had likely been exposed to the remedies of Paracelsus, the anatomy of Vesalius, and the surgery of Paré. When they arrived in America, they had some theoretical knowledge, but it held no therapeutic advantage in curing the natives. European physicians were talking about medical principles but not curing those patients in need. Traumatic injuries may have been the exception to this rule (Table 3.5).

The details of therapeutic advances included in the European pharmacopoeias utilized by European-educated physicians in early colonial America had not fully described specific treatments. Their information was frequently obtained from indirect writings referring to the practicing physician of the times. Botanicals were a good portion of their pharmacopoeias. Sophisticated treatments were rare; simple treatments were more common but seldom effective.

Specific Treatments in English Colonial America

With or without formal education, American physicians preferred to use a more aggressive course of treatment. Heroic medicine, as it came to be known, included emetics, cathartics, diuretics, diaphoretics, and various other evacuants such as antimony, calomel, niter, and ipecacuanha. Opium and frequent bleedings completed the physician's therapeutic repertoire. Bleeding was thought to help rid the body of the disease that was causing the illness. On the contrary, bleeding only weakened the patient and could even lead to death if the patient was too weak or the bleeding too voluminous. Despite the risks, some patients did seem to get better, and thus the practice of bloodletting continued. Purging or vomiting was also used to help patients suffering from almost any malady. We know today that purging can lead to dehydration and even death in extreme cases. In some cases purging seemed to help, and the treatment with purging went on for some time. The use of cathartics had similar effects on the patient. They were laxatives and were believed to be helpful in cleansing the body of the offending illness. Cathartics, too, can lead to dehydration and intestinal motility issues if used chronically. Again because of their supposed success, they were also used frequently.

Opium was one of the most popular pain relievers of the time, and it was often used during operations. Other methods included alcohol, mandragora, and hyoscyamus. In the late 17th century, Peruvian or cinchona bark, with quinine as the main ingredient, was frequently used to treat fevers in the colonies. Sydenham had already suggested this therapy in England, after the Spaniards had recognized its positive effects in Peru. From Peru, it was brought to Europe around the 1630s. The English first found it in the 1650s, and popularized its use in the British colonies at that time. When Oliver Wendell Holmes (1809-1894) re-examined the role of the physician in colonial America, he noted that their pharmacopoeia contained mainly simple treatments such as St. John's wort, clown's all-heal, spurge, fennel, saffron, parsley, elder, snakeroot, and opium.

Diseases, especially those associated with an infectious source, plagued the English American colonies. In this regard, malaria, yellow fever, typhoid fever, influenza, scarlet fever, dysentery, smallpox, and other infections covered the colonial field. Treatment was non-existent, and the mortality rate reached alarming proportions. Not infrequently, the use of aggressive heroic measures was counter productive and further increased the morbidity and mortality seen with these pathological entities.

As time continued in the life of the colonies, European medical knowledge improved, yet no appreciable progress resulted in the management and treatment of diseases. Medical practice of the English American colonies did not change much as it moved into the eighteenth century. It had been written that "facts discovered in the seventeenth century frequently produced theories in the eighteenth century" (Blanton). Physicians did not possess the appropriate therapeutic arsenal to modify the course of disease. Although medical knowledge in the eighteenth century did differ from that of the early seventeenth century, medicine would have to wait for the nineteenth century to bring more ideas and understanding of disease, which would blossom into effective therapy in the twentieth century.

Conclusion

Indeed, Europeans knew medicine before and during colonial times, but it did not amount to a great deal of practical treatments of diseases. Basic theoretical knowledge did not translate into improvement of therapeutics. Some concepts grasped by the colonial physician resulted in treatments ranging from minimally therapeutic to detrimental. The well-cultivated knowledge of European doctors needed more time to mature into an organized and systematic approach to disease. Great empirical findings were being slowly accumulated to form a well-defined body of knowledge with future important implications for the medical sciences of the next generation.

CHAPTER 4
MEDICINE GETS ACADEMIC*

In the sixteenth century, America's first English-speaking medical schools were not on the horizon when medical education began to flourish in European cities such as Padua, Leyden, London, and Edinburgh. In the era before the advent of American medical schools, physicians' practices in America varied little from those used in Europe. The biggest difference between Europe and British America was the limited number of educated doctors practicing medicine in America. The first medical school in the thirteen English colonies of America was at the University of Pennsylvania, which opened its doors in 1765. Like many medical schools around the world, it was modeled after the best universities of Europe. Although American medicine generally kept pace with the major European advances in teaching and practice, it wasn't until after the University of Michigan medical school opened in 1850 and later Johns Hopkins University medical school in 1893, that American medical education began to compete and emerge from the shadows of its European counterparts.

Medical Education Before Medical Schools

According to Harold B. Gill, Jr., author of *The Apothecary in Colonial Virginia*, as British America was first being colonized in the early 1600s, the Virginia Company offered economic incentives to lure physicians across the Atlantic to where doctors were in scarce supply. However, the doctors who made the voyage were often disappointed to find that most colonists did not have money for the service of a physician or lived too far away from the physician to consult him. So in lieu of learned physicians, colonists resorted to home remedies or sought advice from uneducated men with limited medical skill. *Sickness and*

* Partially published in *J Invest Surg*, 17:3-7, 2004, by Toledo-Pereyra L.

Health in America, edited by Leavitt and Numbers, notes that before 1700, only about 140 men and an undetermined number of women practiced medicine in Massachusetts. Only about 20% of the practitioners were apprentice-trained. Most were without formal education, in great part due to the lack of colonial medical schools. This is in sharp contrast to the situation in England, where between the years of 1603 and 1643, four out of five country practitioners had some sort of formal training.

John Duffy, author of *Epidemics in Colonial America*, states in his book that the medical practices of the early 1700s, including bleeding, vomiting, blistering, and purging, which in conjunction with the large quantity of quacks, contributed to the disrepute of the colonial medical profession. In *From Humors to Medical Science*, Duffy also indicates that the start of formal medical education in America could be dated to 1750. In *American Medical Schools and the Practice of Medicine: A History*, Rothstein says that private courses were the true beginning of formal medical education in America, and they established a "distinction between the theoretical parts of medicine, which were taught in courses, and the practical parts, which were taught by the apprentice system." Duffy adds that the first private course in anatomy was offered by John Bard and Peter Middleton in New York. Anatomy lectures were also given in 1752 by Thomas Wood in New Brunswick, New Jersey, and by William Hunter in Newport, Rhode Island, in 1754 and 1756. In spite of all the private courses being taught, even by 1760, the American colonies had yet to produce a medical school. Later on, courses in anatomy would become the cornerstone of every academic medical school established in the eighteenth and early nineteenth centuries.

Medical Schools in Europe Before 1800

A steady stream of medical students left America to go to European schools from the colonial days onward. These physicians studied principally at London, Leyden, and Edinburgh. They were some of the most famous physicians of their time including John Morgan and Philip Syng Physick from Philadelphia and Benjamin Waterhouse from New England. By the eighteenth century, the Italian university in Padua had lost its prominence as interest in anatomy began to take a back seat to clinical medicine and chemistry.

Edinburgh was becoming the center of the Scottish Enlightenment in the mid and late 1700s as well as the early 1800s. The University of Edinburgh benefited from its ties with Leyden. Leyden was the "leader of European clinical medicine." Many of the best physicians of Edinburgh spent a part of their professional lives at Leyden. Between 1749 and 1800, 117 Americans received their degrees from the University of Edinburgh, usually in postgraduate study. Students at the Edinburgh school studied anatomy, botany, chemistry, materia medica, and the practice of physic.

Origin of the First English-Speaking American Medical Schools

According to Rothstein, the push for medical schools in colonial America grew out of a realization by ambitious young doctors with predominantly European training that degree-offering medical schools with a "physical presence in the community" would "enhance the professional reputations of their faculty" and add "stability" to the profession. Many of these aforesaid doctors approached colonial colleges about starting medical schools in the mid-eighteenth century. Rothstein says that colonial colleges welcomed the addition of medical schools because the medical schools would enhance their reputation. However, in reality, the medical schools had little connection with their colleges except for the awarding of degrees. Colleges and medical schools kept an affiliation between them only because the medical school needed the authority of the college to award degrees and because the college needed the medical school to give the appearance that it was broadening its curriculum.

Medical schools had several advantages over apprenticeship training and private courses. Students liked the medical schools because they awarded degrees, which impressed potential patients more than a preceptor's apprentice certificate. The degree let possible patients know that a physician had the most up-to-date knowledge available. Faculty members benefited from medical schools because being appointed to the faculty of a medical school was a mark of prestige and because the names of the faculty were popularized in school advertisements. This rationale, supported by students and faculty, caused the number of medical schools to increase. Five medical schools (Pennsylvania, Columbia, Harvard, Dartmouth, and Transylvania) opened on a degree-granting basis in the late 1700s (Table 4.1). The number increased considerably to a total of 20 schools by 1825. The majority were located in New England, New York, and Philadelphia. The graduates increased from 221 before 1800 to an estimated 1,375 students in the decade from 1810 to 1819 (Rothstein).

Table 4.1: First American Medical Schools founded between 1765-1799
1. Medical Department of the College of Philadelphia, 1765 (University of Pennsylvania)
2. Medical Faculty of King's College, New York, 1767 (Columbia University)
3. Medical School of Harvard College, 1782
4. Medical Department of Dartmouth College 1797
5. Medical College of Transylvania University, Kentucky 1799 (closed by mid-nineteenth century)

During the early nineteenth century, public and private institutions were both interested in developing medical schools. The academic standards were variable but the social impact of these newly graduated doctors would improve the medical profession. Not all medical schools lasted a great time after their foundation. In Table 4.2 we include the institutions that opened in the early nineteenth century and are still in operation today. Some of them were incorporated under different names than the ones we see today.

Table 4.2: Medical Schools Rooted in Early Nineteenth Century American Medicine and Still Operative Today
University of Maryland, 1807
Yale University, 1810
University of Cincinnati, 1819
University of Vermont, 1822
Thomas Jefferson University, 1824
University of Virginia, 1824
George Washington University, 1825
Medical College of Georgia, 1828

Early Entrance and Graduation Requirements Before 1800

When the first British American medical schools opened, they did not have strict standards for admission. People would buy tickets for admission to lectures open to anyone interested in attending. However, as early as 1767, the medical school at the University of Pennsylvania was already tightening requirements for admission and for graduation. These requirements would later become common practice in the 1800s.

By 1800, standard requirements included knowledge of Latin and natural philosophy. Latin was considered important because of its utility in reading classical medical literature and was used to weed out people who lacked a general education. Natural philosophy was only taught in colleges, so a student would have to have attended college or have been privately tutored in the subject before entrance. But, medical schools made their admission requirements vague and therefore allowed for flexibility in student selection.

In order for a student to graduate from medical school, he was required to be 21 years of age, to certify that he spent three years as an apprentice with a preceptor, to complete two course of medical school lectures (none of which were graded), to pass an oral examination, and in the eighteenth century, to prepare and defend a thesis (Rothstein).

General Teaching Practices in Early American Medical Schools

Most medical schools agreed that the curriculum consisted of seven subjects. These were anatomy, physiology, chemistry, material medica, medicine, surgery, and midwifery. In the early nineteenth century, diseases of women and children were added to the curriculum. Lectures were usually conducted by faculty members reading from hand-written manuscripts. Sometimes, students would see demonstrations in chemistry and pharmacy or watch as ambulatory patients were treated. Occasionally they would even see a minor operation in clinical courses. Teachers emphasized how to practice medicine "such as useful prescriptions and descriptions of natural histories of diseases." There was an extremely limited amount of hospital teaching, which was mostly optional in the few colleges that had hospitals, the first and foremost being the Medical Department of the College of Philadelphia. Clinical training was limited because a student only listened to what a patient had to say and there was no actual contact with the patient.

Early Medical Schools Curriculum, 1800s

The medical school curriculum was divided into scientific and clinical subjects. The scientific subjects were anatomy, physiology, chemistry and natural philosophy, which included parts of physics, chemistry, botany, mineralogy, and zoology. The clinical subjects were medicine, surgery, obstetrics, and diseases of women and children. Materia medica had both scientific and clinical aspects. Anatomy buttressed the curriculum of most medical schools. Anatomy had two parts: lectures and practical anatomy (the dissection of cadavers). This class was often made optional in the early nineteenth century because of the difficulty in obtaining cadavers.

The other basic medical science courses were chemistry and physiology. Chemistry was mostly inorganic and was often taught by non-physicians. Physiology was integrated with lectures on anatomy and the theory of the practice of medicine. It also examined the "vital" properties of the body—"motion and irritability, and the functions of the human organs, such as respiration, locomotion, excretion, and circulation of the blood."

Materia medica combined basic and clinical science. Much of this course involved "describing, identifying, and preparing the ingredients" for botanical and mineral drugs. The course was originally designed for doctors who had to prepare their own drugs, but the course continued to be taught even after commercial drugs became widely available. Materia medica was usually taught together with therapeutics.

Clinical courses were all taught as lectures and were made to supplement the clinical training offered during the apprenticeship. Medicine or the "theory and practice of medicine…consisted of descriptions of the effects of disease on the human organism and the changes produced in the blood, circulation, respiration, digestion, and secretions." These descriptions were not based on actual observation, but on contemporary theories instead. In surgery, future doctors observed minor operations. They were usually performed in front of the entire class. Obstetrics, "which usually included the diseases of women," was "taught with the use of plaster and other models because it was considered indecent to expose a parturient woman to the class."

Highlights of Some of the First English-Speaking American Medical Schools

The Medical Department of the College of Philadelphia, 1765

There were only two medical schools in the British American colonies before the American Revolution (1775-1789). The first medical school program opened its doors in 1765 and was the Medical Department of the College of

Philadelphia, today the School of Medicine of the University of Pennsylvania. The second was the Medical Faculty of King's College, New York, which opened in 1767 and is now the College of Physicians and Surgeons of Columbia University (Table 4.1).

According to Edward Potts Cheyney's *History of the University of Pennsylvania 1740-1940*, the actual introduction of medical courses into the curricula of the Medical Department of the College of Philadelphia took place in 1765. In *Medicine at Harvard: The First Three Hundred Years*, Beecher and Altschule indicate that Philadelphia was a "fitting place for such a venture, because in 1765 it was the largest town in the North American Colonies." It was also fitting because it was quickly growing economically as a seaport and as a merchant area. Besides that, Philadelphia already boasted the first successful hospital in the colonies, the Pennsylvania Hospital built in 1750.

Dr. John Morgan (1735-1789) (Figure 2) was the founder of the medical school and its first official professor of medicine. He graduated from the College of Philadelphia and apprenticed with Dr. John Redman. Redman was a well-respected doctor in Philadelphia who had received his MD at Leyden in 1748. While working with Redman, Morgan served for a year as apothecary in the then-new Pennsylvania Hospital. After the completion of his apprenticeship, Morgan obtained a military medical commission and gained some surgical experience with troops in the campaign of 1759. He spent the following year studying medicine and observing in London hospitals under such men as John Fothergill, William Hewson, and John and William Hunter. In 1761, Morgan entered the University of Edinburgh. At Edinburgh, Morgan met an old classmate named William Shippen, Jr. (1736-1808) (Figure 3). Morgan and Shippen discussed a plan to begin teaching medicine at Philadelphia. After his graduation in 1762, Shippen returned to Philadelphia and gave the first formal medical lectures in the English colonies. Morgan received his degree in 1763 from the University of Edinburgh and traveled to France and Italy where he listened to medical lectures and visited hospitals. He was elected Fellow of the Colleges of Physicians of Edinburgh and London, and of the French Royal Society of Surgery, and was made a Fellow of the Royal Society (in London) soon after. During his travels he had developed a plan of introducing a medical college into the American colonies. According to the University Archives and Records Center at the University of

Pennsylvania, Morgan used the University of Edinburgh as his model and chose to build the medical school within an existing college. The early faculty of the medical school earned their medical degrees at the University of Edinburgh and added to their knowledge base with further studies in London. Because the faculty had their hospital experience in London, they chose to stress the importance of supplementing medical lectures with bedside teaching at the Pennsylvania Hospital (Figure 1). The first faculty of the school was made up of Morgan, who taught botany and the practice of medicine; William Shippen, who taught anatomy, was also professor of surgery; William Smith, who taught natural and experimental philosophy; and unofficially, Dr. Thomas Bond, who taught clinical medicine. Two years later, Adam Kuhn joined the faculty and was appointed professor of botany and materia medica. The year after that, Benjamin Rush (Figure 4) began to teach chemistry at the medical school. The first students of the Medical Department of the College of Philadelphia graduated in 1768, two years after the school had opened. The total enrollment in 1768 was only about forty students. Between 1768 and 1774 the College of Philadelphia awarded twenty-nine MB (Bachelor of Medicine) degrees and five MDs. During this same time period King's College awarded only twelve MBs and two MDs.

Medical Faculty of King's College, New York, 1767

King's College was the first school to give the degree of MD in English America. According to *A History of Columbia University 1754-1904*, Dr. Samuel Clossy, a graduate of Trinity College in Dublin, began giving lectures in anatomy in 1763 at King's College before the medical school was founded. Four years later, Clossy and five other physicians (John and Samuel Bard, Peter Middleton, James Smith, and John Jones) proposed creating a medical school modeled after the universities of Great Britain within the already existing King's College. In 1767, the Board decided that a medical school would indeed be established. Unlike the medical school in Philadelphia, King's College was not as much interested in "physic," what we would call internal medicine, as it was in surgery. When the school opened, Samuel Clossy served as professor of anatomy, Peter Middleton as professor of physiology and pathology, James Smith as professor of chemistry and materia medica, Samuel Bard as professor of the theory and practice of physic, John Jones as professor of surgery, and John V. B. Tennent as professor of midwifery. David C. Humphrey's *From King's College to Columbia*

1746-1800 mentions that "professionals" such as Middleton, Clossy, and Bard looked down upon "empirics" and structured the school's curriculum around their belief that professionals should be taught to be scientific and ethical. They admired the "rational physician" who "organizes his medical knowledge into theories which explain the functioning of the body and the cause and treatment of disease." Instead of using a previous treatment or trial and error for unusual sickness, he "applies the ideas he had already formed in his mind, about the nature of diseases in general, to this particular case; by which he easily discerns the genius of the disease; whence it arises; the true indications of cure; and what method ought chiefly to be pursued." *A History of Columbia University 1754-1904* says that the first baccalaureate (Bachelor of Medicine) degrees went to Robert Tucker and Samuel Kissam in 1769. The same individuals earned the first doctorates in 1770 and 1771. Nine other people received their baccalaureate degree by 1774, and thereafter the degree was terminated.

Medical School of Harvard College, 1782

The Medical School of Harvard College opened its doors in 1782. According to Beecher and Altschule in their book *Medicine at Harvard: The First Three Hundred Years*, the proposal for a school was first made at the meeting of the Boston Medical Society of November 30, 1781. It happened when Dr. John Warren (1753-1815) was asked to repeat a course of anatomical lectures similar to those he had given the previous year at the military hospital. Warren suggested that since there seemed to be an adequate number of students wanting to attend lectures, a medical school should be established. It just occurred that at the same time, Harvard College began to think seriously about setting up its own medical school. A committee was organized to discuss the matter and responded favorably. The committee described the establishment of professorships of physic at the college. Professors were to be elected and confirmed by overseers.

Harvard had three professors at its opening. The first was John Warren (father of John Collins Warren (1778-1856) of surgical ether anesthesia fame). He was appointed the first professor of anatomy and surgery on November 22, 1782. He felt that "the greatest needs were for systematic instruction and clinical experience." Shortly thereafter, Benjamin Waterhouse of Newport, Rhode Island, was appointed Professor of the Theory and Practice of Physic, and Aaron Dexter was named Professor of Chemistry and Materia Medica.

The Medical Institution of Harvard College was officially open on October 7, 1783. The school was modeled after the University of Edinburgh; its initial surgical practices were especially influenced by this connection. Medical students at Harvard would attend formal lectures for a semester or two and then were apprenticed to a practicing physician for several years. They weren't required to have any academic preparation prior to coming to Harvard nor were they required to take written exams. The school's first students bought tickets for lectures instead of paying tuition. Harvard did not have a hospital, and as a result, medical students weren't required to have clinical training.

Medical Department of Dartmouth, 1797

Nathan Smith wrote a letter to the Board of Trustees at Dartmouth on August 25, 1796, in which he proposed that a medical school be founded the college. In that same letter, he also told them that if they would establish a medical school and give him an appointment in it, he would study the medical practices of Edinburgh and London and bring that knowledge back with him to teach to Dartmouth medical students. Smith went to Edinburgh for three months and then went on to London where he also spent three months, researching the practices in the Edinburgh and London hospitals and schools. Shortly after his return, Dartmouth Medical School opened in 1797, still without board sanction. Nathan Smith, who is considered the founder of Dartmouth's medical school, was the first to give medical lectures there in that year. It wasn't until 1798 that the board of trustees established a one-man professorship in chemistry and materia medica, anatomy and surgery, and the theory and practice of physic. That same year, the school also established a curriculum which closely followed that of Harvard. Nathan Smith taught everything virtually alone until 1808 when he invited Alexander Ramsay to lecture on anatomy. Sadly, Ramsay only lasted through one course of lectures at the school. Nathan Smith went on teaching alone after that, always keeping up with the newest medical advances, and the medical institution continued to prosper. Smith did a good deal of teaching at the bedside and often took students with him to see patients. It wasn't until 1810 that the school hired another professor, Cyrus Perkins, to be Chair of Anatomy and to take up some of Smith's duties. In 1812, Smith worked out the requirements for the school to have an MD degree instead of an MB. In 1813, Nathan Smith left the school he had founded to get another one up and running: Yale Medical School.

College of Medicine of Maryland, Baltimore, 1807

The College of Medicine of Maryland was established in 1807. Drs. John Davidge, James Cocke, and John Shaw planned the medical school. Davidge, who became the college's first dean, had trained in Edinburgh and Glasgow, Cocke studied at Guy's Hospital in London and at the University of Pennsylvania, and Shaw had studied at the University of Pennsylvania and at Edinburgh. Davidge gave lectures on practical anatomy and did dissections, surgery and midwifery, while Shaw lectured on chemistry. Cocke also lectured on anatomy and did dissections. In 1848, it would go on to become the first American medical school to institute a residency-training program.

Medical Institution of Yale College, 1810

The Medical Institution of Yale College was still in the planning stages in 1806. It wasn't officially founded until 1810, and didn't open until 1813. Nathan Smith of Dartmouth fame introduced the study of surgery to Yale, and he gave lectures on the theory and practice of "physic," surgery, and obstetrics. Smith was "known for his innovative practical approach" to medicine and surgery. The first faculty members of Yale also included Knight, professor of anatomy and physiology; Benjamin Silliman, professor of chemistry and pharmacy; and Eli Ives, professor of materia medica, botany, and diseases of children. Silliman went on to have an "international reputation as a chemist, textbook author, and founder and editor of the American Journal of Science (1818)." Ives went on to become the first American physician to teach a course in pediatrics.

University of Michigan Medical School, 1850

In Midwestern America, the University of Michigan, established in 1817, was the most prominent American university of the time. They began their medical program in the mid-1800s with the medical school admitting its first class in October of 1850. Abram Sager and Silas Douglass played an integral part in the establishment of the medical school at the University of Michigan. Sager was the first dean of the University of Michigan medical school and also the first professor of the theory and practice of medicine. In 1850, he became professor of obstetrics and later became chair of diseases of women and children. Sager is credited with doing the first Caesarian section in Michigan in 1869. Silas Douglass, who would later become the third dean of the medical school, started out as a professor of chemistry, mineralogy and geology. Later he was asked to teach toxicology and pharmacy (materia medica). Moses Gunn was the third faculty member appointed to a position at the medical school. Gunn was made professor of anatomy and surgery in 1849, before the school had officially opened. Gunn served as dean of the school from 1858-1859. Corydon Ford took over the post as professor of anatomy after Gunn left. Ford wrote several significant works such as "Questions on Anatomy, Histology and Physiology, for the Use of Students." Alonzo Palmer became professor of pathology and the practice of medicine in 1860. Palmer wrote several articles and books that contributed to the study of medicine such as *Homeopathy, What Is It?: A Statement and Review of Its Doctrines and Practice*. In the early 1860s, he foresaw in this work the challenge of homeopathy to regular medicine.

Johns Hopkins University Medical School, 1893

In spite of some real advances in medical education, medical schools were not pursuing research in general as an important part of their educational mission. In the late nineteenth century, Johns Hopkins University attempted to do that. According to Richard H. Shryock's book *The Unique Influence of the Johns Hopkins University on American Medicine*, Daniel Coit Gilman, the first president of Johns Hopkins University was inaugurated on February 22, 1876. Shryock notes that Gilman modeled the university after the best institutions in Britain and Germany, and he modeled the new Hopkins Hospital after Guy's Hospital in London. Gilman planned both the university and the hospital a full decade before they opened. He was advised by several respected European and American doctors, particularly William H. Welch, in regard to the training of medical students at the new university.

Early appointments to the faculty of Johns Hopkins Hospital included William Welch, who was very familiar with German medical institutions, as Pathologist-in-Chief (1884) and Canadian William Osler, who was knowledgeable of British medical institutions, as Physician-in-Chief (1888). Other members of the original faculty, all highly respected in their fields, included William Halsted in surgery and Howard Kelly in gynecology. In 1893, John

Jacob Abel was appointed in pharmacology, Franklin Mall in anatomy, and William Howell in physiology. By then, the whole medical school was fully organized and beginning to show some promise.

What made Johns Hopkins so revolutionary was its integration of teaching and research and its drive to get the best doctors of the time on its faculty. That it had small classes, real clinical teaching, and laboratories in the basic sciences made it stand out as well. The school also sought to give attention to new fields that were virtually ignored by other American medical schools such as mental illness, pediatrics, public hygiene, and medical history.

Conclusion

Since the first American medical school opened in 1765, American medicine and medical teaching practices have followed some of the European models of education with apprenticeship remaining an essential part of medical training. Leyden, Edinburgh, and London were prominent models of European descent that were influential in the development of English American medical schools. On this continent, Pennsylvania, Columbia, Harvard, and Dartmouth were the American heirs of European medical genesis. Other schools in the mid-nineteenth century such as the University of Michigan founded medical departments to prepare medical students to a better way of medical practice. With the advent of schools based more in the German system such as Johns Hopkins University, the introduction of dedicated and full-time faculty physicians, and the inclusion of courses in anatomy and dissection, America began its own unique and distinguished path developing the world's best medical schools.

CHAPTER 5
AND NOW WE CAN PUT THEM TO SLEEP

The discovery and use of ether for general anesthesia for surgery was an eminently American contribution to medicine and undoubtedly the greatest development of nineteenth century American medicine. Morton, Wells, Jackson, and Long were the primary players of this extraordinary tale. John Collins Warren (1778-1856), the chief surgeon at the Massachusetts General Hospital in Boston, used ether for the first time in 1846, under Morton's direction (Figure 5); Wells mitigated pain with nitrous oxide in his dental office in Hartford, Vermont; and Long had utilized ether in his hometown of Athens, Georgia. All of them were great contributors that fostered the development of ether for surgical anesthesia. To tell the saga of the American conquest of pain is not an easy undertaking since multiple players, quarrels and disagreements originated from this unique discovery. Hereforth, we give a historical description of the management of pain in general and discuss how the United States of America made its special mark on the medicine of the world.

Brief History of Pain Control

The history of pain relief can be traced back to ancient times. A variety of substances have been used throughout the years to dissipate pain. The Greek physician Dioscorides gave mandrake to comfort his patient. Mandrake is a plant potion that induces sleep. Dioscorides claimed that mandrake produced "anesthesia," the Greek word for without feeling. This would later become the term for the loss of sensation with or without consciousness. Chinese and Indian physicians used marijuana and hashish. Opium was also widely used in various parts of the world, as was alcohol. Willow bark, which contains salicylic acid, was at times used to decrease pain. Traveling quacks knew the value of distracting a patient's mind when undergoing surgery. This led to experimenting with hypnotism and mesmerism. In his book *We have Conquered Pain*, Dennis Fradin states:

> Surgeons were known to enter the operating room with a bottle of whiskey in each hand—one for the patient and the other for the doctor so that he could endure his patient's screams.

Prior to the emergence of ether, horror stories existed of patients screaming helplessly in pain as doctors did their work. Most patients were reluctant to undergo surgery out of fear of suffering. The main tools of a surgeon in the early 1800s were a scalpel, a bone-saw, boiling water, and gauze, or forceps and a cauterizing iron.

There have been many steps that were necessary to occur before anesthesia could exist as it is known today. In 1275, Raymundus Lullius, a Spanish physician, while experimenting with chemicals, made a volatile and flammable liquid he called sweet vitriol. In 1540, a German scientist wrote of the synthesis of ether. Also in the sixteenth century Paracelsus, a Swiss born physician and alchemist, made chickens breathe sweet vitriol and noted that they not only fell asleep but also felt no pain. Neither of the men ever experimented on humans. The inhalation of vapors was employed to treat a variety of aliments including phthisis, catarrh, asthma, and ureteral colic. Yet, all of these elements were never considered for the treatment of human pain. In 1730, Frobenius gave sweet vitriol its present name, ether, which is Greek for "heavenly."

<u>Other Chemical Advances</u>

In 1772, Joseph Priestley, an English scientist, discovered the gas nitrous oxide. Sir Humphrey Davy discovered the anesthetic properties of nitrous oxide. In 1800, he published *Researches, Chemical and Philosophical, chiefly concerning nitrous oxide*. In this essay, he suggested the possibilities of using nitrous oxide during surgery, based on his painless removal of a wisdom tooth. In a later publication he wrote that nitrous oxide,

> appears capable of destroying physical pain, it may probably be used with advantage during surgical operations in which no great infusion of blood takes place.

His suggestions fell on deaf ears. He was also the man who dubbed the term "laughing gas," as an acknowledgement of the euphoria nitrous oxide induces. His student, Michael Faraday also experimented with nitrous oxide and suggested surgical implications, as well.

In 1794, English physicians Thomas Beddoes and Richard Pearson used ether to treat various aliments including fevers and scurvy at the Beddoes Pneumatic Institute. In 1805, American physicians used ether to treat pulmonary inflammation.

In the 1820s Henry Hickman, who was also an Englishman, conducted several experiments with anesthesia. A medical practitioner and a surgeon, he showed experimentally that carbon dioxide could induce asphyxial narcosis. Hickman sent his work to the Royal Society of London, whose president was none other than Humphrey Davy. The Royal Society was not receptive to Hickman's findings and disregarded him. This was a fortunate event since carbon dioxide was not the correct agent and in fact it would have been very harmful.

Samuel Guthrie (1782-1848) was an American chemist, physician, and farmer. He studied medicine with his father and thereafter attended two courses, one at the College of Physicians and Surgeons in New York in 1810, and the other one at the University of Pennsylvania in 1815. He then settled in New York where he produced choleric ether or chloroform in his chemical laboratories. Shortly thereafter it was discovered in Germany and France. In January 1842, William E. Clark administered ether to a patient while Dr. Elijah Pope, a dentist, extracted a tooth. The act was not publicized and was therefore not acknowledged as significant.

History of Anesthesia—Early Encounters in the United States of America

The history of anesthesia is a rather complicated one since there was no clear-cut discoverer. Several individuals claimed to be the leading pioneer in the introduction of surgical anesthesia. The introduction of anesthesia was the first great medical discovery in the United States. By the mid-nineteenth century, the world was ready for the introduction of anesthesia. The proper technology was available, and there was significant demand. Both a climate of humanitarianism and the incentive for fame and wealth steered this invention. The ignorance of the physician, due in good part to his medical education, was a reason why anesthetics were not employed at the beginning of the nineteenth century. When speaking of anesthesia in the nineteenth century, ether was administered using the "rag and bottle" technique. This consisted of placing a piece of gauze over the patient's nose and mouth and allowing drops of liquid ether or chloroform to drip onto the gauze and evaporate into a mixture of gas and air which the patient inhaled.

Owsei Temkin, noted medical historian, has written, "Sociologists of science have cited in evidence for social causation the multiple appearance of the same discovery, 'multiples' in the language of Robert Merton." The lack of a systematic effort to discover a method to alleviate pain may be explained by the fact that medical research at this time was based on autopsies, where pain is nonexistent. As science and society progressed, the stage was set for the introduction of anesthesia. The demonstration of ether in 1846 led Ulrich Trohler to write, "it can be seen as a heroic landmark in the history of modern surgery."

The work of many scientists and physicians prepared science and medicine for the introduction of anesthesia. By most historical accounts, four major contributors (Long, Morton, Wells, and Jackson) are usually credited with the introduction of anesthesia. These four men helped bring the method into public use.

The first of the contenders for "the father of anesthesia" was Crawford Long (1815-1878). Long was a country doctor in Danielville, Georgia. He studied at Franklin College, which would later become the University of Georgia. He received his medical training at both Transylvania University and the University of Pennsylvania in 1839. While attending medical school, Long engaged in laughing gas parties, also known as nitrous and ether frolics, which were extremely popular. At the time nitrous oxide and ether were used as forms of entertainment. "Chemical lecturers" traveled from town to town, giving nitrous oxide demonstrations at fairs and meeting halls. When Long returned to Georgia to practice medicine he introduced laughing gas parties to the people of his hometown. On one occasion at a laughing gas party, Long offered his friends sulfuric ether as a substitute for nitrous oxide. Long observed as a friend injured his leg without reaction while under the influence of ether. The friend acknowledged that pain existed only after his euphoria from ether had subsided.

Crawford Long recognized the medical implications of this discovery immediately. On March 30, 1842, in Jefferson, Georgia, Long successfully administered ether to James Venable, a medical student, while removing a tumor from his neck. This is the first known use of anesthesia. Two months later Long used ether to remove another tumor from the neck of the same patient. In July 1842, Long painlessly amputated a young boy's toe using ether. Within the next three years, Long successfully used ether on three more patients.

Without a doubt, Long was the first physician to use ether on patients during surgery. The reason why Long is not acclaimed as the discoverer of anesthesia is simple; he neglected to report his findings to the medical community until 1849. He published "An Account of the First Use of Sulfuric Ether by Inhalation as an Anesthetic in Surgical Operations" in the *Southern Medical and Surgical Journal* in 1849. He did, however, obtain affidavits of the efficacy of ether. At the time of his publication there were already other contenders for the title and rewards that accordingly come with being the discoverer of anesthesia.

One of these contenders was Horace Wells (1815-1848) from Hartford, Vermont. Wells was one of the leading dentists in Hartford during his time. In 1844, Wells saw a demonstration of the usefulness of ether by the popular lecturer Gardner Q. Colton (1814-1898), a disciple of P.T. Barnum. During this lecture Samuel Cooley, a participant under the influence of ether injured his leg and did not feel any pain. This mesmerized audience members, including Horace Wells. This experience was very similar to that of Crawford Long. Within a short period of time Wells had resolved to determine what the implications of ether would be on dentistry.

In 1844, with the aid of Dr. John M. Riggs, Wells painlessly extracted one of his own teeth. "A new era in tooth pulling," he is said to have proclaimed. What separates Wells from Crawford Long is that Wells was determined to share his discovery with the rest of the world. In January 1845, with the aid of former dentistry partner William Morton, Wells administered nitrous oxide on a patient before a medical class at Massachusetts General Hospital. This demonstration was set up by one of Boston's leading physicians and medical professor at Harvard, Dr. John C. Warren. Everything in the demonstration went accordingly until the patient unexpectedly yelled out in pain. This caused the class of medical students to boo, and the experiment was determined to be a failure. However, the patient later said that he felt no pain and had no control over his outburst. Regardless of this admission, Wells was utterly embarrassed and returned to Hartford mortified.

The third and most important contender was William Thomas Green

Morton (1819-1868). Morton had dreamed of becoming a physician but did not have the financial means to achieve this goal. Instead, he was tutored by Horace Wells in dentistry in the early 1840s, and for a time in 1843, the two shared a short-lived dental practice. He also practiced dentistry in Charlestown and Boston, Massachusetts. Morton participated in the failed anesthetic demonstration by Wells. Morton claimed to have graduated from the Baltimore College of Dental Surgery; however, research has shown that he never attended medical or dental school. Nevertheless, in 1852 Washington University in Baltimore gave Morton an honorary MD. Morton recognized the amount of pain that existed for patients in his dental practice and began to experiment with different ways to alleviate this pain. He met with Charles Jackson, professor of chemistry and geology at Harvard and the final contender, who suggested that Morton should apply sulfuric ether to the gums of his patients. Morton began working with ether in secret, building on the principles that Jackson had taught him. He experimented with small animals at his estate in West Dedham, Massachusetts. This culminated when Morton administered ether on himself and went into an exhilarated state. At this stage Morton was prepared to make public his findings.

Using the same forum as Horace Wells, Morton planned a demonstration with the approval and support of John Collins Warren, chief surgeon at the Massachusetts General. In the days and, better yet, the hours before the demonstration, Joseph M. Wightman and Nathan B. Chamberlain developed a device to administer ether. Morton and Augustus A. Gould, MD, a physician at the Massachusetts General Hospital improved upon their device. The final product was a sponge, soaked in ether, within a glass container with valves to control the dosage. On October 16, 1846 Morton successfully administered ether as Dr. Warren removed a tumor from the neck of Edward Gilbert Abbot, a man who had come to the Massachusetts General Hospital for the treatment of a vascular tumor on his jaw. This was the first victorious public administration of anesthesia (Figure 5). After the operation, Abbot, replying to questions on whether the procedure had hurt, stated, "No. It didn't hurt at all, although my neck did feel for a minute as if someone were scraping it with a hoe." Dr. Warren is noted to have said, "Gentlemen this is no humbug," and with these words a new era in medicine began. The dome of the Bulfinch Building where the act took place was to become known as the "Ether Dome." In recent years, the administrative staff of the hospital has celebrated Ether Day every year in October to commemorate the introduction of ether to surgical anesthesia.

The Morton/Warren demonstration went so well that the very next day the duo put on another exhibition. Word quickly spread of the incredible feat, and Morton became quite famous in Boston. Dr. Oliver Wendell Holmes, the acclaimed physician-poet in Boston, knew of the Greek physician Dioscorides who had utilized the word anesthesia and recommended the name of anesthesia and anesthetics to Morton. Describing the excitement of the time the *People's Journal of London* stated,

> Oh what delight for every feeling heart to find the new year ushered in with the announcement of this noble discovery of the power to still the sense of pain, and veil the eye and memory from all the horrors of an operation...we have conquered pain.

On November 18, 1846, Dr. Henry J. Bigelow published "Insensibility During Surgical Operations Produced by Inhalation" in the *Boston Medical and Surgical Journal.* The article was the first published account of a successful etherization. The article recounted how Bigelow had witnessed four operations in the previous months, in which Morton administered anesthesia while Dr. John Collins Warren or Dr. George Hayward performed the procedure. This article quickly excited the medical community in Boston, and they gave Morton all of the backing for discovering anesthesia. In 1847, Morton published "*Proper Mode of Administering Sulfuric Ether by Inhalation*" in an attempt to promote his work. Before describing the events following Morton's demonstration the final actor should be discussed.

Charles Jackson (1805-1880) called Plymouth, Massachusetts his home. Jackson spent much of his time dabbling in science, especially chemistry, physiology, and geology. He was also an unknown inventor, a professor at Harvard, and a noted tutor. In 1844, Jackson argued to have had suggested using ether to soothe patient's pain to William Morton. This is Jackson's primary claim to being the founder of anesthesia. Jackson proposed that he was unknowingly aiding a friend, who then used his knowledge and insight against him. Jackson asserted that he was the true discoverer of the benefits of ether and that Morton simply stole what was rightfully his. At the same time that Morton was giving lectures in Boston about the implications of his discovery, Jackson was doing the same. However, Jackson's audiences were less receptive to his claims. In Table

5.1, we summarize the events leading to the successful use of ether in surgical anesthesia.

Table 5.1: Some Historical Events Leading to the Discovery of Ether Anesthesia for Surgical Use		
Year	Individual	Event
1275	Lullius	Use of Vitriol
1500s	Paracelsus	Use of Vitriol
1540	German Scientists	Synthesis Ether
1730	Frobenius	Use of Vitriol
1772	Priestley	Discovered Nitrous Oxide
1800	Davy	Use of Nitrous Oxide
1820s	Hickman	Use of Carbon Dioxide
1825	Chapman	Effects of Ether
1832	Mitchell	Ether Frolics Description
1840s	Miller	Ether Frolics Description
1842	Clark	Use of Ether in Dentistry
1842	Long	Use of Ether in Surgery
1844	Colton	Nitrous Oxide Exhibition
1844	Wells	Use of Nitrous Oxide in Dentistry
1844	Jackson	Suggested Use of Ether to Morton
1846	Morton	Use of Ether in Surgery

Following the use of ether, chloroform became the anesthetic of choice. James Y. Simpson, head of obstetrics at Edinburgh, first introduced chloroform to relieve obstetrical pain in Scotland in 1847. Ether was known to have a bad odor, irritated the lungs, made patients vomit, and had awkward equipment. This led directly to the more frequent use of chloroform, which was quicker, cheaper, more powerful and lasted longer. It should be noted however that excessive amounts of either chloroform or ether was known to produce serious side effects and even death.

Difficulties in Assigning a Single Discoverer

After the various incidents, these pioneering men engaged in a bitter battle of who was the true discoverer of anesthesia. For different reasons, all men had a partial claim. The controversy spread all the way to Congress, the newspapers, and Europe. William Morton, in an attempt to make a profit, created a substance called Letheon. Morton simply added oil of citrus to mask the telltale odor of ether. Adding to the controversy was that the United States granted William Morton a patent, U.S. patent #4848 on November 12, 1846, for his method of etherization, which used a glass jar with a rubber tube. Morton gave up his dental practice to concentrate on promoting Letheon, causing him great economic hardship. Contributing to Morton's state of financial plight was the fact that even the U.S. government would not pay him royalties on his patent. This was demonstrated during the Mexican-American War (1846-1848) when the army used its own inhaling devices without paying Morton a cent. This, in effect, sent a message to surgeons and dentists that it was not necessary to recognize Morton's patent. Several times Congress came close to allocating $100,000 as a reward to Morton. However, the appropriations bill never passed the Senate. When it eventually became clear that Congress was not going to award any of the men any monetary prize for their discoveries, then-President Franklin Pierce urged Morton to sue the U.S. government for $100,000 for its employment of etherization during the Mexican-American War. It was Pierce's belief that this was the only manner in which Morton could be compensated for his efforts. The case remained in the court system until 1862, when the decision was rendered that Morton would receive nothing since what he had patented was a procedure and therefore was unpatentable, a nonsensical attitude in the patent law of today.

Results on the Battle for Supremacy

The battle over credit for discovering the use of ether was not without casualties. Charles Jackson made several attempts to claim priority both in the United States and France. With unconvincing evidence and a less than credible history, Jackson met very little success in his campaign. He had earlier sued Samuel Morse over the invention of the telegraph. He also claimed to have invented guncotton, an explosive. Jackson eventually was committed to a mental asylum, where he remained until his death. It is said that Jackson went mad upon reading Morton's tombstone, which acknowledged Morton as the inventor of inhaled anesthesia.

Horace Wells also attempted to claim priority in Washington, with little fruition. Like Jackson, Wells' life also turned tragic in his attempt to earn credit for his role in discovering anesthesia. Wells privately continued experimenting with forms of anesthesia. Wells soon became addicted to chloroform. In 1848 he was arrested for throwing acid on a prostitute, while under the influence of the drug. Two days later while in prison, Wells committed suicide by severing his femoral artery.

Morton, on account of the priority dispute, was rendered penniless and was constantly on the verge of a nervous breakdown. This is well reviewed by James Thomas Flexner in *The Death of Pain,* which hailed Long as Morton's co-discoverer. Morton died of a stroke in 1868, never achieving the widespread acclaim that he so sought. His headstone does bear a legacy in the inscription by Dr. Jacob Bigelow,

> Inventor. Revealer of Anaesthetic Inhalation. By whom pain in surgery was averted and annulled. Before whom in all time surgery was agony. Since whom science has control of pain.

Crawford Long was the only of these four men to live to see old age. He remained a country physician until his death. Long, in contrast to the others, lived a happy, honest, and decent life. Fittingly, he had never sought to profit from his discoveries. In the South, Long did have many supporters, who proposed that he was the first to introduce surgical etherization.

Final Outcome and Consequences

In general the use of anesthesia was quickly accepted in most sectors of society. Before the end of 1846, ether was administered during surgical procedures in both Paris and London. In England, in December 1846, Robert Liston successfully amputated a limb, pain-free. However, it was not a smooth and seamless road to the anesthesia of today. For instance, a noted Philadelphia surgeon, H.H. Smith commented in 1852 that "I have myself affected by extreme lassitude from breathing the atmosphere…during a prolonged etherization." The clergy initially was opposed to the use of anesthesia, believing that it contradicted God's plan for mankind's suffering. This was especially the case when used during childbirth. The Church believed that misery in childbirth was God's punishment for Eve's transgression in the Garden. On the other hand, William Morton commented "unrestrained and free as God's own sunshine, ether has gone forth to cheer and gladden the earth; it will awaken the gratitude of the present, and all coming generations." However, Morton's comments regarding the public's reaction should not be viewed without bias given his self-promoting behavior.

John Snow was the first professional anesthetist in Great Britain. He worked at St. George's Hospital in Hyde Park Corner, London. In 1847, he invented a portable ether inhaler. The first known instance of ether being applied during childbirth was to Fannie Appleton Longfellow in 1847. Also in 1847, Walter Channing, Dean of the Medical School at Harvard, published a work on *Etherization and Childbirth*, hailing the possibilities of the recent discovery. In 1853, Queen Victoria used chloroform during the birth of her eighth child, Prince Leopold, thereby making it an acceptable practice. This royal validation came at an important point as not everyone was fully convinced of the great benefits of anesthesia.

Pierre Flourens, a nineteenth century philosopher, argued that "with the increasing superficiality of the general training of our doctors, the unlimited use of chloroform may encourage surgeons to carry out complex and difficult operations." This helped to further the argument that the new anesthetic procedure could help patients who otherwise did not have an opportunity to be treated for diseases that might require extensive surgery. Flourens did have a valid point; surgeons were encouraged to perform more complex operations and thereby advanced medical science.

There is a widely held misconception that soldiers were never given anesthesia during the Civil War. This is not the case. By the 1860s opposition to anesthesia was rare in the United States. In 1862, a lecturer at the College of Physicians and Surgeons in New York asserted that "the day is past where the administration of anesthetics in surgical operations is subject for discussion." The benefits that ether and chloroform produced quickly hushed their opponents in the medical debate over their use. Professor J.J. Chisolm summarized the attitude of Confederate surgeons in his *Manual of Military Surgery,*

> The universal use of chloroform to allay the pain of surgical operations is a complete vindication for the utility of this remedy, and proof of its necessity...We do not hesitate to say that it should be given to every patient requiring a serious or painful operation.

During the course of the war, Union records showed that at least 80,000 operations were done using anesthesia and only 254 were completed without. Clearly, the use of anesthetics was an accepted practice.

During the Civil War, the pioneers of anesthesia were serving in various military capacities. Morton served as a volunteer battlefield anesthetist for the Union. He eventually attended more than 2,000 soldiers. He took an average of three minutes to administer anesthesia to a fallen soldier on the battlefield. On the opposing side, Crawford Long was in charge of the Confederate hospital in Athens, Georgia. Long had the foresight to order enormous amounts of ether and chloroform, which proved instrumental in the many operations that he performed during the war. By this time, in the mid-1860s, chloroform was the most frequent general anesthetic used (in an approximate scale of five to one when compared to ether).

In spite of the overwhelming use of anesthetics by the time of the war, it was not until the 1870s that anesthesia was a constant fixture in the medical arena. This lack of complete acceptance occurred for several reasons. Many doctors thought that the use of anesthesia brought the patient too close to death. It was also a widespread belief that pain was a necessary part of the healing process. Some physicians believed that the use of ether or chloroform was not natural, which fed off the popular appeal of irregulars and homeopaths.

The debate over who should receive credit for the introduction of anesthesia was never truly resolved. In 1864, the American Dental Association deemed Wells as the discoverer of anesthesia, and in 1870, the American Medical Association followed suit. In 1877, Dr. J. Marion Sims published "*The Discovery of Anesthesia*" in the *Virginia Medical Monthly* journal. It was the first work to acknowledge that all four men had together substantially contributed to the discovery of anesthesia. Perhaps, this is the most accurate account. Crawford Long was the first to use a new process. Horace Wells was the first to advocate widespread use in a populous area and made Boston more receptive for William Morton who made anesthesia an accepted part of medicine. Finally, it is undeniable that Charles Jackson's suggestions were vital to Morton's success.

<u>What Has Been the Impact of the Introduction of Anesthesia?</u>

Today people have the opportunity to receive painless surgery. With the emerging acceptance of the germ theory of disease and ensuing antiseptic and aseptic methods developed in the 1870s, more complex surgeries would become possible. John Galbraith Simmons describes the climate of the time best,

> Surgery reinvented itself in the late nineteenth century. While advances in physiology and pathology made it possible to understand the architecture and some of the dynamics of the human body, anesthesia and asepsis made it plausible to open it up and repair it.

It took many decades for anesthetics to advance to what is now known in the twenty-first century. Even into the early 1900s, the specialty of anesthesia still consisted of dripping ether via a soaked sponge into a patient's nose. Little attention was given to vital signs during the operative procedure until in 1895 when Harvey Cushing noticed the high rates of ether overdose. After blaming himself for the death of a patient due to excessive anesthesia, Cushing and an associate developed the anesthesia record or "ether charts." Following his initiative, blood pressure, pulse, and respiratory rate began to be monitored.

By the end of the first half of the twentieth century, the profession of anesthesiology required four to five years of graduate education after medical school. Today, because of the immeasurable benefits of anesthesia, each year in the United States alone, millions of surgeries are being performed with the administration of anesthesia. There is no question that because of the discovery of anesthesia, society now has the benefit of medical and dental procedures without fear of pain, a luxury that generations past never dreamed possible.

Conclusion

The introduction of ether anesthesia for surgery in the mid-nineteenth century was an American discovery. Four men contributed to this unique experience. William Morton first publicly demonstrated the benefit of ether at the Massachusetts General Hospital on October 16, 1846. The surgery was carried out by John Collins Warren, chief of surgery at the institution. Surrounding the Boston development was the second contributor, Horace Wells, who demonstrated to Morton the techniques of anesthesia and the successful use of nitrous oxide in dental cases. The third player was Charles Jackson who, according to his own account, provided the idea of using sulfuric ether to Morton. Finally, the fourth person was Crawford Long, a general practitioner from Georgia who utilized sulfuric ether for the first time in surgery in 1842 but did not publish or publicly introduce its use. Regardless of the controversy surrounding its origins, the discovery of ether clearly opened an enormous gate in the medical sciences, one that allowed a great number of patients to receive the benefit of surgery without the fear of pain.

CHAPTER 6
NOT ONLY REGULAR DOCTORS CURE

At the beginning of the nineteenth century, the practice of medicine in the young American nation had no consistent therapeutic modalities. In spite of the development of the five medical schools at the end of the eighteenth century, school-educated doctors did not have a great advantage over apprentice-trained physicians. No effective therapy was available. The main manner in which medicine was being practiced was called Heroic Medicine, which consisted of the use of extraordinary measures such as extensive bleeding, vomiting, purging, cupping, blistering, and sweating for the treatment of a great number of illnesses. There was no discrimination of the patient's age, sex, or condition. The type of disease made a difference; the more serious the disease, the more intensive the heroic measures undertaken. Clearly the patient was the hero in accepting these treatments. The purpose of this section is to analyze the reasons for the development of irregular doctors as well as the various schools that originated from this movement.

Reasons for the Development of Irregular Doctors

The medicine of early nineteenth century United States was not providing good medical results. It was far from perfect and a great mortality was evident throughout the whole medical spectrum. The most significant reason for stimulating the appearance of irregular doctors was the presence of Heroic Medicine. With the advantage of the passage of time, almost two centuries afterwards, we can conceive that irregulars were flourishing when regular doctors were showing their poorest results with the heroic treatment of diseases. The public, in general, perceived this enormous difference in results and consequently abandoned the use of regular doctors as their primary caregivers. It was not hard to figure it out, even then, that the use of bleeding for a great number of diseases was not conducive to improving results.

Some of the leading orthodox American doctors such as Benjamin Rush (1745-1813) had learned from their European counterparts and applied the heroic principles with religious commitment to the chagrin of their patients. It is well known that General George Washington, at the beginning of the nineteenth century, succumbed probably more as a consequence of heroic medicine than his alleged bacterial laryngotracheitis infection, not a good example to show to future generations of physicians!

Other factors of important consideration in the rise of irregulars (Table 6.1) were the decline of the prestigious orthodox physicians as well as the return to the egalitarianism of the Age of Jacksonian Democracy, where every man returned to the simple days of early American society and became self-sufficient in every walk of life.

The Age of Heroic Medicine

The age of heroic medicine in the United States of America flourished in the first half of the nineteenth century. The practice of bleeding was usually the preferred treatment. Patients who sought medical help for anything from smallpox to dysentery would normally be relieved of a few pints of their blood. This was done through venesection, scarification, and/or cupping. Venesection was the drawing of blood by opening a vein. Scarification differed from venesection in that the scarification method required a series of small cuts produced by a spring-loaded instrument. The cupping method of bleeding was done with a warm glass container, which allowed the inside atmospheric pressure to drop. The cup would eventually fill as the outside pressure and inside pressure reached equilibrium.

The father of American medicine or American Hippocrates, as he was called so many times, Benjamin Rush, was the most ardent supporter and champion of bloodletting throughout the United States. Dr. Rush was an adamant believer in bleeding as the most reliable way to achieve recovery for a patient. Patients were bled often and with abandon. Rush taught his medical students persistence; if one pint didn't work, then take two or three. When a patient's symptoms did not appear to be subsiding, his students would continue to bleed the patient until he or she either miraculously recovered or died. The bleeding treatments continued even if four-fifths of a patient's blood had already been drawn. This was particularly important and of enormous consequences considering that Rush believed the human body contained twelve quarts of blood, twice the actual amount.

Table 6.1. Development of Irregular Medicine Movements in the United States of America in the Nineteenth Century

Type of School	Main Proponent(s)$^{\Delta}$	Year of Establishment
Homeopathy	Hans Gram, New York	1825
	Constantine Hering, Pennsylvania	1835
	Samuel Hahnemann, Pennsylvania*	1848
	Ruben Leidlam, Illinois	1852
Eclectic-Reformed	Wooster Beach, Kentucky	1831
Botanical	Constantine Rafinesque, Kentucky and Pennsylvania**	——
Thomsonian	Samuel Thomson, Massachusetts***	——
Botanic Medical	Alva Curtis, Ohio	1839
Reformed	Thomas Morrow, Ohio	1840
Eclectic-Botanical	Thomas Cooke, Pennsylvania	1840
Osteopathy	Andrew Taylor Still, Missouri	1892□
Chiropractic	Daniel David Palmer, Iowa	1897•

*Hahnemann did not personally participate in the development of the school, Hahnemann Medical College of Philadelphia, but his name was lent for the naming of the school.

**Rafinesque did not found a school in spite of his enormous influence in the Botanical movement.

***Thomson, like Rafinesque, did not establish a school of medicine even though he contributed extensively to the irregular movement.

□American School of Osteopathy opened in Kirksville, Mo in 1892.

•Palmer School and Cure opened in Davenport, Iowa in 1897.

$^{\Delta}$Life spans of some of the distinguished members of the irregular group: Hahnemann (1755-1843), Ludlam (1831-1899), Beach (1794-1859), Rafinesque (1784-1841), Thomson (1769-1843), Curtis (1797-1881), Still (1828-1917), Palmer (1845-1913).

It is difficult to determine the exact number of unnecessary deaths that could be attributed to bloodletting. Many patients did not recover after severe and frequent bleedings. As mentioned before, George Washington died after willingly opening his veins to Dr. Rush's disciples. Rush wrote of Washington's death in his diary, "This day died, universally lamented, George Washington. His disease was cynanche trachialis. It proved fatal in 14 hours. He was patient and resigned in his illness...He wished his physicians to enable him to die easy..." Washington's illness may have eventually taken his life. However, his bleeding of nine pints of blood in a twenty-four hour time span did not help in this situation. Washington, like countless others, became another patient/victim of the bleeding method of heroic medicine.

Blame for the hurried deaths of so many Americans cannot only be placed on the practice of bleeding. Blistering was also commonplace in the late eighteenth and early nineteenth centuries. Placing hot plasters on the patient's skin would produce a second-degree burn where the plasters had been. The presence of pus, which was drained from the developed blisters, was seen as a sign of recovery from infection.

Purgatives were used in both minimal and massive doses to clean the system. Calomel (mercurous chloride) was the most commonly used purgative. Calomel worked as a simple laxative when prescribed minimally, but when used in high doses, which was common, it would completely purge the system. As one can imagine, these treatments could be horrifying to patients of the time, as well as they are today. The sick and injured of eighteenth century America did not always welcome the heroic treatments (Table 6.2).

Volney Steele, dedicated Montana historian and practicing physician, accurately reviewed the role of the physician on the American frontier. He emphasized how Meriwether Lewis and William Clark "were the first healers from the so-called civilized part of the United States to come to the western frontier." They both had had some medical experience in the army. Meriwether Lewis, in particular, at the request of President Jefferson, had spent some time in Philadelphia receiving direct instruction from the illustrious medical teacher medical teacher Benjamin Rush. Clark had mostly obtained practical medical knowledge on his own. During the long and arduous expedition or "Voyage of Discovery" from 1803 to 1806, Lewis and Clark applied every single medical concoction and procedure available throughout this heroic national enterprise. Everything was valid under these extraordinary circumstances. After all, their accomplishments were impressive. Steele put it very well when he said, "that the group [of around 50 men] suffered only one fatality is miraculous considering the difficulties and dangers of the long trek." An incredible feat!

Table 6.2. Type of Treatments Used by Regular and Irregular Physicians in the First Half of the Nineteenth Century

Type of Treatment	Regulars	Irregulars
Bleeding	Yes	No
Purging	Yes	Rarely (Except for Thomsonians)
Emetics	Yes	Rarely (Except for Thomsonians)
Cupping	Yes	No
Blistering	Yes	No
Herbs/Botanicals	Rarely	Yes
Homeopathy	No	Yes – Homeopathy School
Steam Baths	No	Yes – Thomsonian School
Minerals	No	Yes – Eclectics/Reformed
Exercise, Fresh Air, Cold Showers, Diet of Fiber and Vegetables	Sometimes	Yes – Mainly Sylvester Graham School*

*Sylvester Graham (1794-1851) was a prime supporter of a moderate way of life which included the use of the elements before exposed. He was a key figure in the popular health reform movement.

New methods of treating unhealthy patients soon began to gain favor with American citizens. The concept of Jacksonian democracy would help to push these new irregular treatments and medical theories to the public. Jacksonian democracy was not just a political term. It spread its influence over nearly every aspect of American life. The concept that a man was capable of accomplishing nearly everything that he put his mind to symbolized the ideas of the time period. The citizens of America began to be more self confident of their abilities. The elitist culture that had run Europe for centuries had begun to fade away in the United States. With the new trends in culture, came new trends in the way of life for people in the young nation. Individualism became a sign of the times. People sought to do their own business the way that best suited them. One of the areas that saw the largest change was American medical practice. As never before, Americans searched for new ways of treating their ailments. Several alternatives such as new schools of irregular medicine caught on and gained acceptance as the Jacksonian era unfolded.

Schools of Irregular Medicine

Homeopathy

Homeopathy, a treatment of illness based on the idea that "*like cures like* (*similia similibus curantur*)," was formulated by a German physician of profound intellect and cultivated mind, Samuel Christian Friedrich Hahnemann (1755-1843). Hahnemann was the first person to systematically study and perform true Homeopathy, even though others like Hippocrates had written ideas very similar in nature during ancient times. Paracelsus also studied and wrote about procedures that used likeness to help cure certain illnesses and ailments.

Hahnemann, did not gain his credibility through practicing the medicine he preached. Although he did serve as a practicing physician, he never opened a homeopathic clinic. In fact, Hahnemann gave up the practice of medicine in 1779, the very same year he received his medical degree from the University of Erlangen. After leaving medical practice, he began to work as a translator and soon began writing commentary on medical practices. He wrote his first published essay, "*Directions for Curing Old Diseases*," in 1784. That work and the ones that followed gave medical advice on nutrition, good hygiene, and exercise. Hahnemann continued to do research and writing on topics such as arsenic poisoning, syphilis, and cinchona bark in the years that followed. It was his work with cinchona and its medical impact which would help spur his theory of homeopathy.

Cinchona bark, "Jesuits' bark," as it was coined, had been brought to Europe from Peru. Hahnemann did not agree with the accepted medical beliefs on why cinchona helped to reduce fevers. In order to better understand how cinchona affected the human body, Hahnemann began testing it on himself. He administered it orally twice daily. Noting the side effects on himself, Hahnemann found that cinchona produced cold extremities, quickened pulse, headache, dry mouth, and other symptoms common of a fever.

Hahnemann soon began testing other plants and drugs on himself. He then moved on to studies on other patients. His testing on others was done basically the same way as his self-testing. The patient would take the medication, wait, then write down or describe to him the effects that were felt. After doing his research, Hahnemann wrote his *Essay on a New Principle for Asserting the Curative Powers of Drugs* (1786). In this paper, he first referred to his concept of *like cures like* as homeopathy.

Homeopathy was based on two main doctrines, that of *like cures like* and the law of infinitesimals. This second doctrine declared that by diluting a drug after the third time to a millionth of a grain, the patient would receive the greatest possible benefit. Later on, he would recommend further dilutions to the thirtieth dilution. According to Hahnemann, the patients who were given these infinitesimal amounts experienced improved results. He was very careful about not exceeding the doses suggested, otherwise he felt the patients could be injured. He never explained the reasoning behind the homeopathic concept. This was a completely new concept but without any substantiation. Hahnemann believed he had found a new law of nature.

These radical new concepts set homeopathy apart from mainstream physicians or "allopaths" as Hahnemann called them. Despite the tremendous differences between accepted medicine and homeopathy, the method began to spread. When compared to many common medical customs such as bloodletting and purgatives, homeopathy was a non-painful alternative to many people. Retaining their blood and not being subjected to burns, cuts, and vomiting appealed to many of those seeking medical attention. Because of this, homeopaths enjoyed greater success than the regular physicians' heroic maneuvers during successive cholera epidemics that began in 1832.

The practice of Homeopathy first began in Germany and other parts of Europe. The United States was extremely receptive to all new ideas. By 1825, Hans Gram, an American born of Danish parents who obtained his medical degree in Copenhagen, introduced the benefits and value of the practice of Homeopathy in New York City. New Yorkers without much difficulty began to embrace this fresh new doctrine. John F. Gray, a disciple of Gram, started his own practice of Homeopathy in 1828 in New York City. Many other physicians followed Homeopathy as a response to this new trend in medicine (Table 6.1).

In 1835, Constantine Hering, a distinguished German physician and scientist, emigrated to Pennsylvania, where he established the Allentown Academy, the first homeopathic college in the United States of America. Other important colleges of this sort, like the Hahnemann Medical College of Philadelphia, would not be founded until 1848.

While homeopathy did enjoy growth as its concepts took hold in the conscience of Americans, it also received a great degree of criticism. Many mainstream physicians were writing and speaking out against the new system of medicine. One of these doctors who spearheaded the movement against homeopathy was the well-known physician, poet, and medical educator, Oliver Wendell Holmes (1809-1894). Holmes and his fellow skeptics attacked the two main doctrines of homeopathy. The law of infinitesimals caught a great deal of flack from the Boston physician/poet. When he studied the law, Holmes came to a conclusion. If a druggist were to carry out his homeopathic preparations to the seventeenth dilution, it would take the contents of "ten thousand Adriatic Seas," to prepare the medication correctly. Holmes used this example along with many others to help curb the excitement built up by the masses. His 1842 lecture to the Massachusetts Medical Society, *Homeopathy and Its Kindred Dillusions*, began a nationwide movement of discussions on homeopathic credibility. In spite of the enormous sense made by the logical conclusions of Oliver Wendell Holmes, regular physicians did not have anything new and better to offer. Thus, the practice of Homeopathy continued on.

The organization of the American Medical Association (AMA) in 1847 presented a more consistent opposition to irregulars. The development of the first code of ethics by the AMA gave a decided disadvantage to the becoming groups of non-regulars. In the years that followed, homeopathy reached new heights as it referred to the development of new homeopathic hospitals, colleges, and local and national organizations. Kaufman, noted medical historian specializing in *Homeopathy in America*, summarized extremely well the status of this field in the classic book *Other Healers*, edited by the recognized historian Norman Gevitz. In this work, he indicated:

> By 1844, there were enough homeopaths around the country to establish America's first national medical society, the American Institute of Homeopathy...By 1860, there were a total of 2,399 homeopathic physicians in America with 699 in New York, 325 in Pennsylvania, 207 in Massachusetts, 188 in Ohio, and 158 in Illinois...By the 1880s there were homeopathic medical colleges in most major cities, including Boston, New York, and Philadelphia. At the University of Michigan both homeopaths and allopaths were educated, with allopathic professors teaching everything to students who intended to practice orthodox medicine, and homeopaths teaching homeopathic therapeutics and materia medica to students intending to practice homeopathy.

In the 1920s, there was a renovated interest for improving medical education in the country, particularly led by the Flexner report, which had appeared ten years before. This critical study condemned all substandard medical colleges which gave a reason for eliminating all poor schools. Among them were most of the homeopathic colleges. Only four homeopathic schools stood up; Boston University, Hahnemann Medical College of Philadelphia, New York Homeopathic Medical College, and the University of Michigan. In 1922, the homeopathic department of the University of Michigan was eliminated, when the amalgamation of the allopathic and homeopathic departments took place. The rest of the 1900s was not hospitable to the re-organization of the homeopaths. Fewer potential members wanting to support this movement became available. By the 1960s, homeopathy had practically disappeared because of the practicing physicians being over the age of sixty. As the century advanced, the alternative health movement gave some new enthusiasm to the homeopathic school of medical thought. Still, organized orthodox medicine did not fully accept homeopathy within its own ranks. Meanwhile, since 1980, the Arizona legislation established a homeopathic licensing board, and three years later, classes began for a three-year term degree of homeopathy at the Arizona Homeopathic Medical University College of Medicine in Scottsdale. Other states such as California, Florida, and Georgia are following in the steps of Arizona's initiative.

Botanical Medicine

Botanical medicine offered a wide variety of opportunities for those physicians interested in the use of plants or herbs in the treatment of disease. It included many forms and methods of practicing medicine such as Native American remedies, Thomsonianism, and herbal therapies. Since mainstream medical treatments could also include some botanical remedies, this created a difficult division to make between irregulars and regular practitioners.

The Native Americans of the initial thirteen colonies and the British settlers were both interested in the use of plants and herbs. The Native Americans had better access to the major botanical sources for the treatment of disease. As British colonists and settlers made the trip west across the Atlantic, medical plants made their way east to Europe. Substances such as guaiacum, sarsaparilla, balsam of Peru, lobelia, cascara sagrada, cocaine, curare, capsicum, arrowroot, cocillina, jalap, and tobacco all found their way into European medical kits. These new found plants with medicinal qualities would soon make a great impact on European medicine. In turn, American medicine would also change in years to come.

Herbal and botanical mixtures now joined the mineral and metallic laden medications that had dominated the medical world. In America, doctors soon began studying and implementing these new botanical medicines. Constantine Smaltz Rafinesque (1784-1841) is considered the Father of the Botanical School of Medicine in the United States. He was a Frenchman living in Constantinople who came to the American continent for the first time in 1812 and returned in 1817. At this time, he became professor of botany at Transylvania University. A few years later, he moved to Philadelphia where he published his most important work, *Medical Flora; or Manual of Medical Botany of the United States of North America* (1828-1832). This book represented the book to consult for physicians practicing botanic medicine in the United States. Other physicians, such as Christopher Witt, John Bartram, and Benjamin Smith Barton, also participated in developing this new field. It was their dedicated work that led to another form of alternative medicine. As time went by, the botanical movement lost popularity and by the twentieth century few physicians were adhering to this school of practice.

Thomsonianism

Samuel Thomson (1769-1843) was an uneducated farmer from Cheshire, New Hampshire. His parents were strict Baptists who only owned their property on credit. Being raised poor and in a rural setting shaped Thomson's experiences and had a profound effect on his adult life.

One aspect of Thomson's youth that influenced his life was the informal medical attention that he received growing up. Living in the countryside of New Hampshire made it virtually impossible to visit a trained physician. Instead the family got their medical advice and treatment from a local widow by the name of Benton. The widow Benton grew close with Samuel during his childhood. Often she would take him along with her in search of botanical and herbal medicines. The pair would walk the local woods searching out various types of plants. On their trips together Thomson was taught many of the names and uses of the local plant life. On one of his walks, Thomson came upon a plant that was new to him. He quickly went about consuming the plant and found it to have an emetic influence on him. In the years that followed, Samuel used this plant (*Lobelia inflata*) for his own enjoyment. He would convince his friends to eat the plant as he had, and then he would sit back and watch as they would quickly grow ill and vomit. Thomson continued to use his "emetic herb" eventually using it on a local farmer. The normal outcome, vomiting, occurred. However, this time the man who had consumed the Lobelia saw a quick improvement in his overall health. After witnessing his "patient's" health improve, Thomson concluded that he possessed "a gift in healing the sick." He now set out to create a method for his style of medicine.

Other important and influential events in the life of Thomson included the death of his mother, which he blamed on the use of mercurials and other heroic medicine products, and the treatment of his wife with the frequent use of bleeding and other severely injuring therapies. These unpleasant experiences tainted his appreciation of regular medicine and made of him an ardent supporter of herbal medicine. As early as 1805, he became an itinerant herbal practitioner, depending mainly on the use of botanicals and steam baths.

Thomson had a very simplistic approach to disease. He formulated his therapeutic principles on a poor understanding of some of the Greek medical treatments. He insisted that there was only one disease, produced by cold, and one cure, enacted by the use of heat. Thomson, then, believed in overcoming the cold by using steam baths and similar measures that reinstituted normality or the presence of warmth.

Additionally, Thomson adopted the ancient idea that all animal bodies were based on four elements: earth, fire, air, and water. Thomson wrote that "Earth and water constitute the solids, and air and fire, or heat, are the cause of life and motion." He used these four elements of life as the guidelines for his practice. In order to keep patients alive or to better their health, he would have to make certain that they did not have a lack of heat. When the body lacked or lost all heat, the patient would then die. He then set out to gain more knowledge on the plants, minerals, and herbs that would aid in keeping the essential heat.

While collecting specimens and gaining experience, Thomson decided it would be necessary to record his data. He wrote, "I deemed it necessary that whatever discoveries I should make in my practice, they might be so adapted to my plan, as that my whole system might be easily taught to others, and preserved for the benefit of the world." Overall, Thomson created a new alternative form of medicine, Thomsonianism. Thomson also conveyed his ideas and recommendations in a book published in 1822, entitled *New Guide to Health; or Botanic Family Physician.*

Another aspect of Thomsonianism was based on the use of six different vegetable medicines. Thomson withheld their specific names; fittingly they were then named Number One through Number Six. Each medicine contained more than one herb or vegetable, except for Number One. This medicine was the same plant as he had discovered as a young boy, *Lobelia inflata*. He used this to clean out the stomach (through vomiting) of anything that could deplete the body of its essential heat. Thomson concluded that something as simple as drinking an excessive amount of cold water could lead to death. Thomson felt that when the body lost its internal heat such as "by throwing into the stomach so large a quantity of cold water as to give the outward heat the power of balancing the inward," one could succumb to death.

Thomsonianism did not only attempt to rid the stomach of unwanted matter, it also saw already digested material as a problem area. Thomson gave his patients enemas in order to remove fecal matter that he felt could be harmful. He used bitterroot, bayberry, and slippery elm in his enemas. Each of these were used after he had tested them upon himself. He would continue to use both purgatives and enemas until he felt the body had been rid of its imbalance.

If neither purgative or enema found the desired results, or sometimes in addition to their use, Thomson would steam his patients. This was done in the way of a crude sauna with the addition of eating cayenne pepper. The main desire from steaming the patients was their perspiration. This was thought to rid the body of unwanted imbalances. Both the steaming and the ingestion of cayenne were thought to help promote the patient's heat.

The steaming portion of Thomsonianism did not remain in favor as the method spread throughout America. The vegetable medicines soon began to take over as the preferred method of home practitioners. This can be accredited to both the excessive time and extra materials needed for steaming.

The easy access to the medicines used, and the inexpensive costs of them led to the widespread enthusiasm of Thomsonianism. Thomson recommended that, "every family to have on hand a stock of medicines that included one ounce of the emetic herb, two ounces of cayenne, one to two pounds of bayberry root bark in powder form, one pound of poplar bark, one pound of ginger, and one pint of Rheumatic Drops." His followers were quick to follow his instructions and stocked their homes with items found in nearby fields and woodlands. These inexpensive medicines led to the continued growth of Thomsonianism.

Eventually a licensing board and Thomsonian colleges were set up. However the status of Thomsonianism soon went on a steady decline after Samuel's death in 1843. Arguments amongst his followers began to split up the group. By the 1850s, the Thomsonianism movement as a whole was quickly fading into nothing more than cult status.

Eclectic-Reformed

Wooster Beach (1794-1859) was the founder of the Reformed (Eclectic) System in the United States. A native of Trumbull, Connecticut, he did an apprenticeship under Jacob Tidd, a German botanical physician. It is unclear if he obtained an MD in New York after Tidd's death. In 1829, Beach became the first president of the Reformed Medical Society of the United States, and in 1831, the first recognized college of the Reformed School was opened in Worthington, Kentucky. Unfortunately, this college did not last for more than twenty years. Beach, like Thomson, began emphasizing the role of botanical products. The Eclectic or Reformed members differed from Thomsonians in their willingness to use other non-botanical means (such as minerals and others) in the treatment of diseases.

Other schools of irregular medicine included the Botanico-Medical School sponsored by Alva Curtis from Ohio, the Reformed School supported by Thomas Morrow from the same state, and the Eclectic-Botanical School championed by Thomas Cooke from Pennsylvania (Table 6.1). Many other movements would appear and disappear in the course of the nineteenth century. By the end of the nineteenth century, many schools of irregular medicine were no longer actively practicing

Phrenology

Another alternative form of medicine that climbed its way into the culture of Jacksonian America was the science/art of phrenology. This practice was brought to America from Great Britain, where it had first gained success early in the nineteenth century.

In America, phrenology was spread by the Fowlers, a family who dedicated themselves to the practice and preaching of phrenology. The Fowlers began their lecture and head reading tours in New York in the 1830s. From New York they eventually spread throughout New England and eventually to the rest of the United States.

The practice of phrenology was essentially the reading of the bumps and contours of a patient's skull. This was done with either the tips of the fingers or the palms of one's hands. Occasionally, a measuring tape was needed for proper reading. It was first thought that someone's brain or "mind" could be mapped out during a reading. While doing the reading, a phrenologist would advise his patient on what type of occupation they were best suited for, what type of spouse they should marry, what foods would be best to eat, and what types of activities they should partake in.

Phrenologists related to both mental philosophy and human physiology by making four basic assumptions. First, the brain is the origin of the mind. Second, the specific faculties are located in specific parts of the brain. Third, each part of the brain holds a specific faculty. Fourth, the brain's size and shape determine the size and shape of the skull. The first two assumptions hold some validity today. We look at the brain as being our mind, not just part of our mind. Modern research has shown that specific areas in the brain do represent certain functions within the body.

The popularity of phrenologists can be credited to the fact that they did not just stay in one specific location. Many phrenologists traveled around the country spreading their ideas and providing their service. By going out to the country fairs, farmers' markets, and other community activities, phrenologists spread their ways to the masses. It should be noted that long after phrenology had lost its appeal to much of the urban American population in the post-Civil War United States, some rural Americans still were willing to spend their hard-earned money for the services of a phrenologist. At the turn of the last quarter of the nineteenth century, the phrenology movement had very few followers and was completely by the twentieth century.

Osteopathy

Andrew Taylor Still (1828-1917) is the father of osteopathy; he conceived on his own an unique and distinctive system of medical care which consisted in the use of musculoskeletal manipulation, particularly of the spine, to cure disease due to "obstructions inhibiting the flow of blood and nervous fluid" (Numbers).

Still grew dissatisfied with orthodox medicine, especially after the death of three of his children in 1864. Homeopathy and eclecticism did not convince him either. He considered internal medication immoral and at some point in his life he was attracted by magnetic healing and bonesetting. His most important discovery was that flexion and extension procedures of the spine were a better means of healing than any other procedure. Misplaced bones of the spine were the source of disease and unbalance.

In 1892, Still began the American School of Osteopathy in Kirksville, Missouri. This school saw the education of a great number of noted osteopaths. Four years later, Still strengthened the curriculum of the school by increasing the time of study to four terms of five months each and by adding physiology, surgery, theory, and practice of medicine and midwifery to anatomy and osteopathic principles already being taught. In 1897, plans to establish the American Osteopathic Association were completed. Osteopaths then had an important forum in which to present their ideas and plan of action.

In the first part of the twentieth century, bills began to be enacted in the legislation in an increased number of states that favored the osteopathic movement. Eamons Booth (1851-1934) in a classic report described by Gavitz, intensely expressed his deep concern about the present two-year curriculum. As a consequence a three-year plan was suggested and accepted. Several schools had reservations about this policy, and some of them closed or merged. By this time, there were four thousand DOs (Doctor of Osteopathy) in practice. By 1915, DO colleges in Boston, Chicago, Des Moines, Kansas City, Kirksville, Las Angeles, and Philadelphia were the only recognized active schools in the country.

By 1916, the DO school requirements had been lengthened to four years, being then equivalent to the number of years required for an MD. The preprofessional needs to enter a DO school were still very different than an MD school in that DO physicians did not require a high school diploma for acceptance. In the 1920s things changed, and this situation was corrected to include high school graduation for all applicants. By the 1930s all schools were compliant in this regulation.

In 1940, osteopaths, not satisfied with their current preprofessional requirements, adopted a two-year college compulsory regulation. By 1954, three years of college were required, and six years later, almost three-quarters of the accepted class had a bachelor's degree or higher. Osteopathic medicine had reached a comparative level to orthodox allopathic medicine, and for practical and legal matters, they were equivalent. In 1969, with strong support from the legislation, Michigan State University accepted the first university college of osteopathic medicine. This unique school operated in the same building occupied by the College of Human Medicine. In a very special and unique way, both osteopath and allopath schools worked together effectively, and in this way osteopathy left the field of irregulars to enter orthodoxy in a complete and successful manner.

Chiropractics

In September 1895, Daniel D. Palmer (1845-1913), a Canadian schoolmaster and entrepreneur who had practiced magnetic healing for a decade, single-handedly developed the use of chiropractic techniques. Later on, in 1910, Palmer said, "I created the art of adjusting vertebrae, using the spinous and transverse processes as levers." Years before, in 1902, he founded the first school of Chiropractics in Davenport, Iowa, the Palmer Infirmary and Chiropractic Institute. The origins of this school go back to 1896 when Palmer incorporated the Palmer School of Magnetic Cure, and in 1897 he renamed it the Palmer School and Cure

Several important personalities participated in the progression of chiropractic principles and therapeutic contributions. B. J. Palmer (son of the founder), Solon Massey Langworthy (according to Russell Gibbons, the first to establish a systemized curriculum), Minora Paxson, Oakley Smith (the last three chiropractors co-authored the first chiropractic book published in 1906, *A Textbook, Modernized Chiropractic*), Andrew Davis, William Carver, John Howard, and William Schulze were among the best examples of the profession.

Chiropractors continued their ascent to gain recognition in the United States. By the 1970s, after frequent legal battles and multiple antagonistic positions from orthodoxy or regular practitioners, governmental agencies, the public, and organized medicine began accepting chiropractics as a profession with a defined scope and specific indications. Chiropractors concentrated their attention on spinal manipulation, and thus their filed of expertise was well-defined and not impinging upon regular MDs (Table 6.3).

Table 6.3. Other Important Medical Information About Some Irregular Medical Schools During the Nineteenth Century

Irregular School or Movement	Founder	Origin	Based	Book/Other	Important findings
Thomsonian	Samuel Thomson (1769-1843)	US	▪ Botanical, herb medicine ▪ Use of heat and cold ▪ Attacked all regular medicine	▪ "New Guide to Health" ▪ Development of Friendly Botanical Society ▪ 1840: NY support legislation ▪ 1848: Licensing boards in Connecticut ▪ 1827-1891: 22 botanical medical schools founded	Use of Lobelia Inflata as emetic
Homeopathy	Samuel Hahnemann (1755-1843) Hans Gram Constantine Hering John Gray	Germany Germany, US Germany, US US	Law *"similia similibus curantur"* (like cures like) (e.g. cinchona)	*Organon* (book) same disagrees with book same	▪ Tests of drug: "provings" ▪ Length of effect and dose ▪ Recommended 30th dilution ▪ Two schools: high and low dilutionists ▪ Zenith US: 1880
Graham Movement	Sylvester Graham	US	Exercise, good food, right living	None	N/A
Osteopathy	Andrew Still and many others	US	Musculoskeletal manipulation	*Journal of Osteopathy*, *Osteopathic Physician*	In late twentieth century, move to integrate with orthodox medicine
Chiropractic	D. D. Palmer	US	Spinal adjustments	*A Textbook, Modern Chiropractic* (1906) *Research Status of Spinal Manipulative Therapy* (1975)	Studies in progress to define benefit of spinal manipulation

Other Irregular Movements

Christian Science Healing

The founder of Christian Science in the United States was Mary Baker Eddy (1821-1910) from Concord, New Hampshire. She was not a healthy individual and suffered from multiple ailments including colds, fevers, lung and liver abnormalities, backache, nervousness, and depression among many others. Unsatisfied with the poor results of orthodox medicine, she began utilizing various irregular treatments associated with Christian beliefs. She called her teachings Christian Science and concentrated most importantly on the significance of strict moral behavior and exclusive commitment to the Bible and *Science and Health.* These last two words represented the title of the first book of Christian Science published in 1875 by Eddy and her disciple Richard Kennedy. This book was the essence on which this movement based its philosophical and practical ways of existence.

By 1910, according to Schoepflin, historian of the Christian Science movement, there were more than 50,000 members associated with this group. From this time forward, the numbers began to dwindle until less than 3,000 members were registered in 1985. It would appear, then, that this movement had reached a precarious position from which little influence could be sought. Christian Science leaders have not give up on their interest to search for increased membership in the years to come.

Other Movements

Several irregular movements from time to time have occupied the attention of various motivated groups in the United States. Since the nineteenth century, skepticism for routine methods to cure the ill has stimulated the development of challenging ideas and a plan of action totally different from what organized medicine had to offer at the time.

Divine Healing has been one such movement. Believing in the healing power of prayer, relying on the providence of God, and establishing places (faith or healing homes) where the word of God could be combined with other healing modalities represented the basis for this new way of seeing and curing the sick.

Spiritual involvement in healing was an important development of the nineteenth century and something that was particularly special to the Pentecostal movement of the twentieth century. The Assemblies of God, the Church of God, and many other sects represented the main tenets of the Pentecostal movement. Healing through divine intervention was the fundamental principle upon which all these organizations sustained their roots. The relationship with scientific medicine was a contentious area of disagreement since most of these groups rose to prominence by exalting committed divine participation in the cult of the ill.

The classic Pentecostal revival movement after World War II was divided into two groups, a moderate one represented by Oral Roberts, who was in favor of a combination of medicine and divine healing, and a more radical movement integrated by A. A. Allen and Jack Cohen, who repudiated medicine and doctors. As time advanced, in the 1960s, radical and conservative ministers preached frequently to similar audiences who were not as responsive as audiences of previous years.

By 1985, American healing revivalism still had a presence in the country, but with a considerably reduced influence. Oral Roberts, on the other hand, had clearly succeeded in amalgamating medicine and prayer, uniting medicine and divine healing, and in developing a new Protestant theology of divine healing. A few years back, in 1975, Roberts stunned his audiences when he proposed and fully built a new medical school and large hospital and research medical center in Oklahoma. With his actions, he was accepting modern medicine although with the use of prayer and spiritualism to improve patient care. Modern Pentecostals by then had already accepted the principles and the best of medical sciences.

Folk medicine in the United States has included an increased number of health traditions and beliefs deeply based on the vast ethnic fabric of the country. From old medical practices represented by primitive cures on the one side and more sophisticated ways of patient care such as Ayurveda and acupuncture on the other side, folk medicine has offered many other alternatives to curing sick. Let's begin with religious folk healing where religion and healing have been closely associated. By definition, all religious beliefs about health and cure are part of folk medicine. In this regard, the Order of Saint Luke (interdenominational), the pilgrimage and the cult of the saints (Catholic), and the psychics healing traditions and the Powwow practices (German and Native American) have represented significant variants of religious folk healing.

Another alternative movement has been natural folk healing. In this group, folk herbalism with its vehicle, the health food movement began searching for a means to modify regular medicine. The Seventh Day Adventists have been at the forefront of this development. They utilized well-organized plans to draw the public attention towards the importance of good living, healthy food, and exercise in the improvement of the health of this nation. At the end of the discussion, the health food culture and folk herbalism had many things in common and many similar religious tendencies as well. For instance, Adventists accept that natural healing has certain closeness to a religious outlook. Also, other movements related to Eastern spirituality, for example, have close ties to folk herbalism and health food.

The complete assimilation of folk medicine into organized regular medicine is not entirely possible. There are some elements in folk tradition that will have a difficult time in gaining full acceptance by regular allopaths. In this case, a point of understanding or communication between regulars and irregulars with the idea of utilizing the best of each one would be in order. Recognizing the social and cultural background of folk medical practitioners would facilitate a greater acceptance of their methods and ideas into the main stream of organized medicine.

The field of alternative medicine is so extensive that this chapter does not attempt to cover all and each one of the health movements associated with it. Its importance is so critical to current medical thinking that under mandates by the U.S. Congress, the National Institutes of Health established an Office of Alternative Medicine in 1991. For those deeply interested in this significant topic, the very well-presented and researched books of Norman Gevitz, editor of *Other Healers: Unorthodox Medicine in America* published in 1988 and the one by James Whorton on *Nature Cures: The History of Alternative Medicine in America* published in 2002 are highly recommended as the most comprehensive and authoritative books on the subject.

Conclusion

Several schools of irregular medicine grew in nineteenth century United States as a consequence of the harsh Heroic Medicine practiced by regular physicians. This consisted of bleeding, vomiting, purging, cupping, and blistering. The age of Heroic Medicine flourished in the first half of the nineteenth century. At one point or another, a great number of regular physicians utilized heroic methods in the country. The results of Heroic Medicine were dismal, with high mortality and morbidity associated with it. This environment cleared the way for irregulars to successfully introduce the practice of irregular medicine.

The irregular movement was represented by the schools of Homeopathy, Eclectic-Reformed, Botanical, Thomsonian, Botanico-Medical, Reformed, Eclectic-Botanical, Phrenology, Osteopathy, Chiropractics, and others. Many personalities were the leaders of this irregular practice of medicine. In this country, Gram, Hering, Beach, Rafinesque, Thomson, Curtis, Morrow, Cooke Still, and Palmer were some of the major leaders. In Europe, Hahnemann was the founder of Homeopathy.

The discussions and debates that arose over each of the irregular methods forced mainstream allopaths to take another look at their methods of medicine. Eventually, around the 1850s, each of the alternatives lost strength both in credibility and in practicing members. Mainstream medicine that was available when the alternatives faded was far from the heroic medicine that had led so many to the irregular doctors. By the 1890s, a great number of the irregular sects had practically disappeared from the world of American medicine, and exceptional examples such as Osteopathy and Chiropractics were to grow into the fields of organized and orthodox medicine.

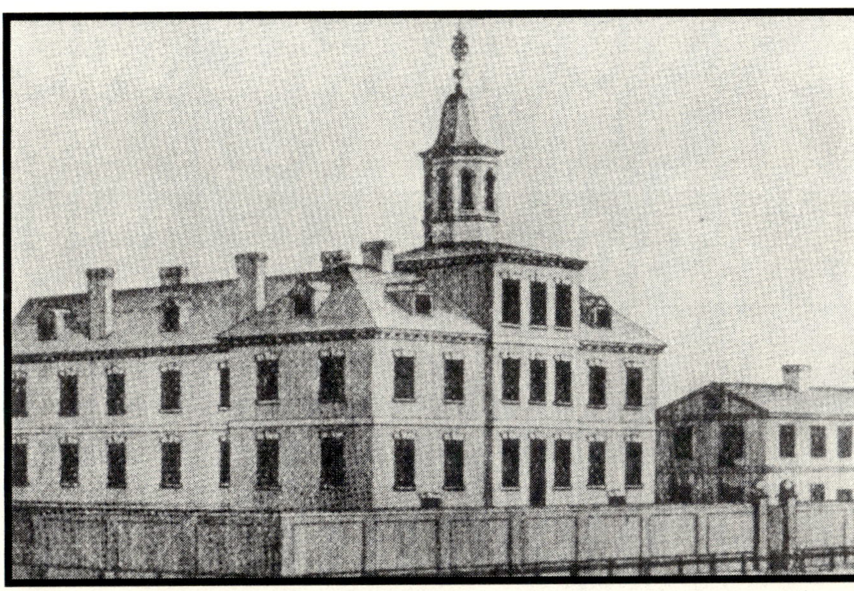

Figure 1. Pennsylvania Hospital, founded in 1751 by Benjamin Franklin and Thomas Bond, was the nation's first hospital. (Engraved by R. Scot, from the Bradley Collection, College of Physicians of Philadelphia; obtained from Bell WJ Jr. *John Morgan: Continental Doctor*. Phildalephia: University of Pennsylvania Press; 1965.)

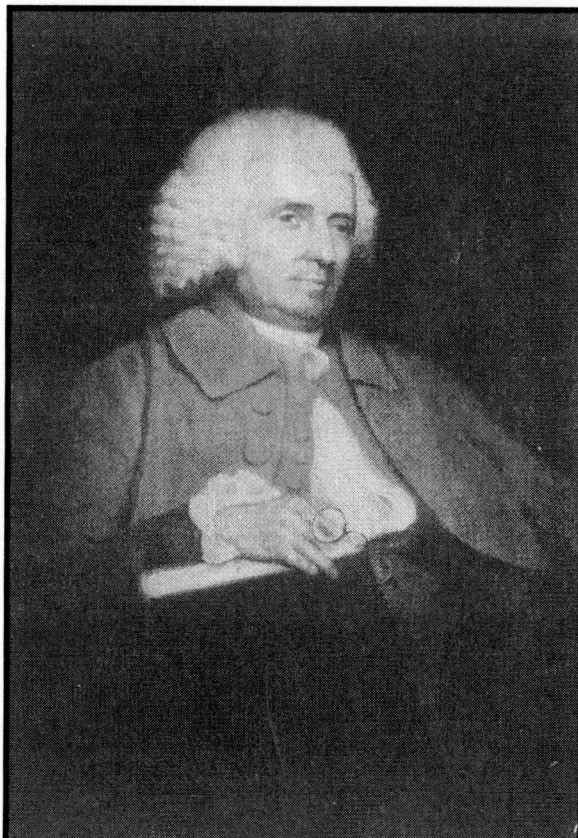

Figure 2. John Morgan (1735-1789), founder of the first medical school in colonial America (1765), the National School of the College of Philadelphia, today the University of Pennsylvania. (Engraving by Thomas Spence Duche circa 1787; obtained from Bell WJ Jr. *John Morgan: Continental Doctor*. Phildalephia: University of Pennsylvania Press; 1965.)

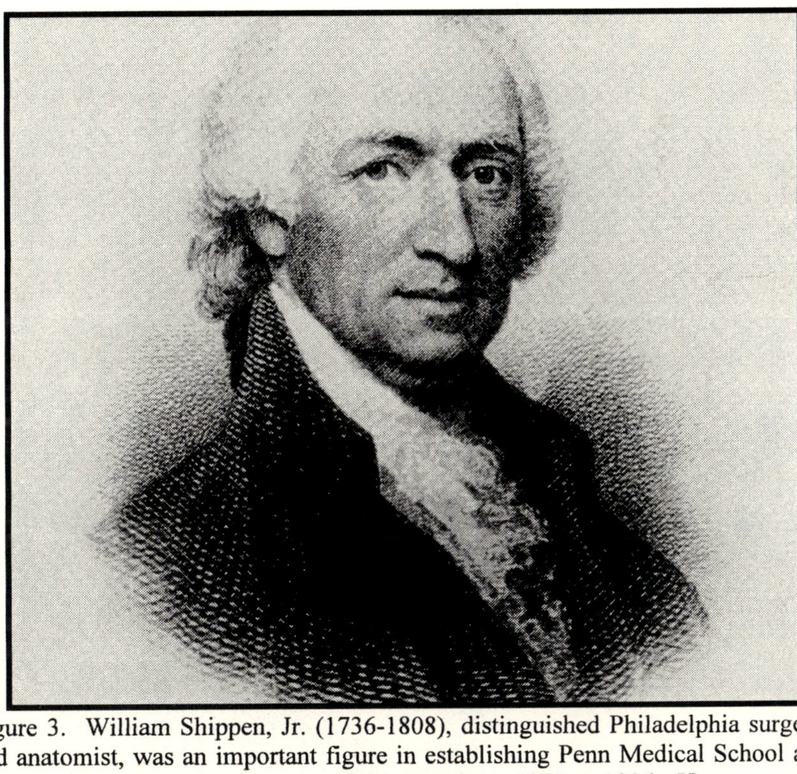

Figure 3. William Shippen, Jr. (1736-1808), distinguished Philadelphia surgeon and anatomist, was an important figure in establishing Penn Medical School and served as Professor of Anatomy and Surgery from 1774 to 1806. He was one of the founders and president of the College of Physicians of Philadelphia. (Engraving of a painting by James R. Lambdin after Gilbert Stuart; obtained from Bell WJ Jr. *John Morgan: Continental Doctor*. Phildalephia: University of Pennsylvania Press; 1965.)

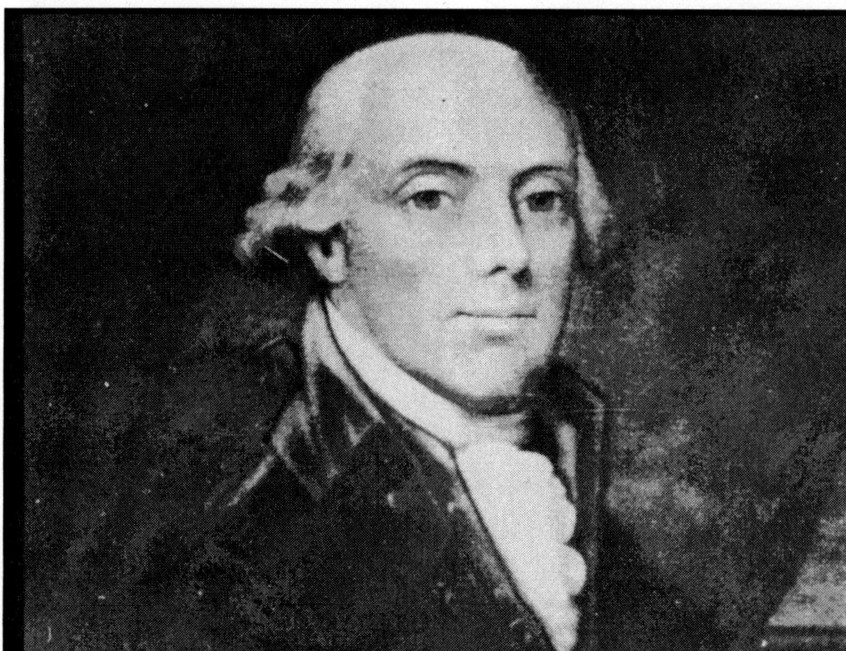

Figure 4. Benjamin Rush (1746-1813), eminent physician of revolutionary America, was one of the earliest contributors in chemistry and *materia medica* to the newly established Pennsylvania Medical School. He is considered to be the Father of American Medicine. (Engraving by Edward Savage from the Bradley Collection, College of American Physicians of Philadelphia; obtained form Bell WJ Jr. *John Morgan: Continental Doctor*. Phildalephia: University of Pennsylvania Press; 1965.)

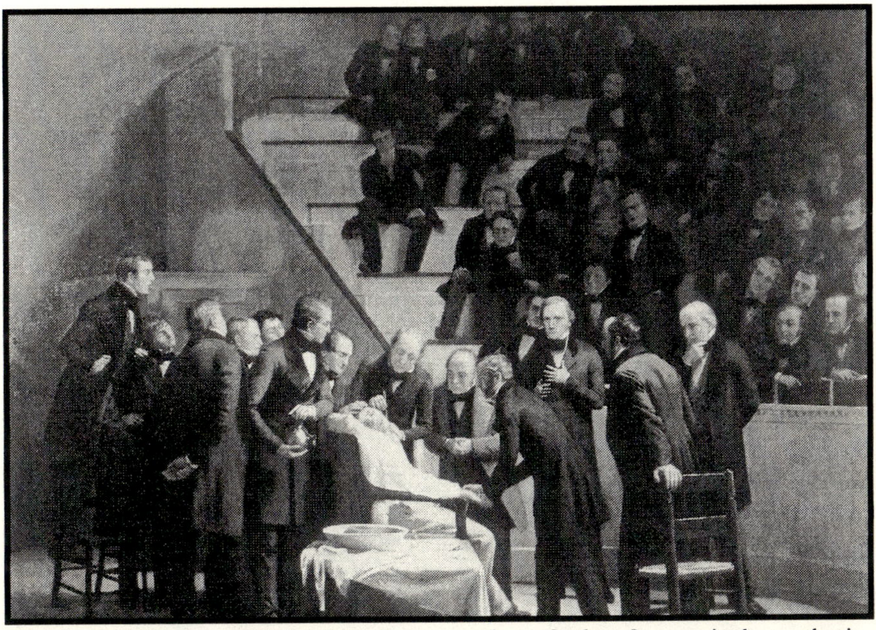

Figure 5. First successful public demonstration of ether for surgical anesthesia, October 16, 1846, at the Massachusetts General Hospital in Boston. (Painting by Robert Hinkley, 1882, currently maintained at the Francis A. Courtway Library of Medicine, Harvard Medical School, Boston, MA; obtained from Lyons S and Petrucelly II RJ. *Medicine: An illustrated history*. New York: Harry N. Abrams Inc.; 1978)

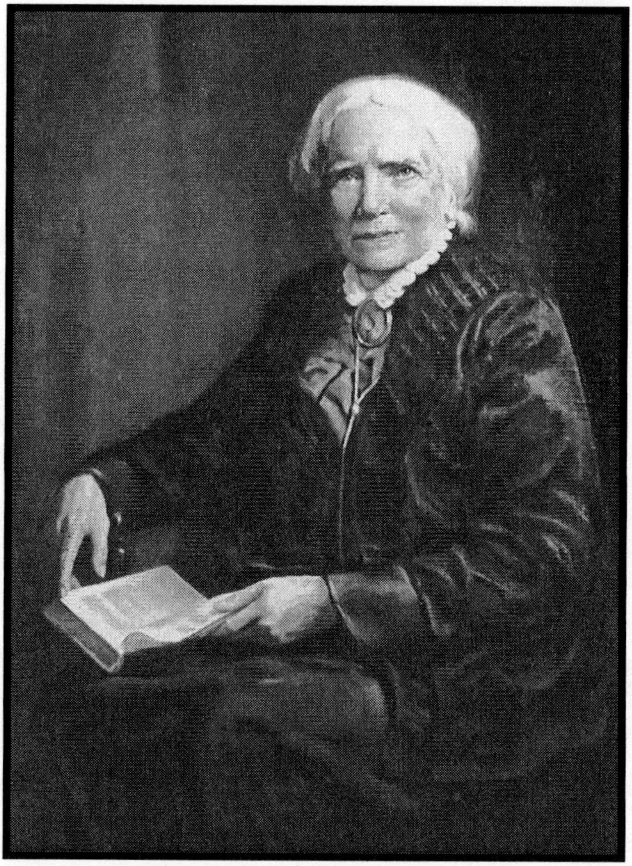

Figure 6. Elizabeth Blackwell (1821-1910), the first woman to receive an MD from an American Medical School, Geneva Medical College, today the Upstate Medical School in the State of New York (1849). The portrait was commissioned by the medical student sorority Alpha Epsilon Iota, and painted by Joseph Stanley Kozlowski in 1963. (Obtained from http://www.upstate.edu/library/history/blackwelloz/jpg)

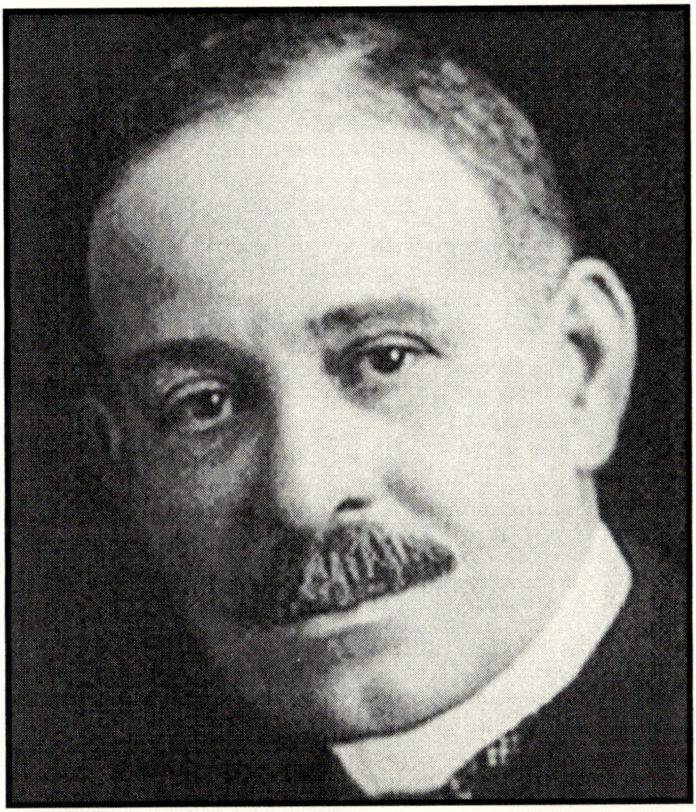

Figure 7. Daniel Hale Williams (1856-1931), pioneering African-American surgeon and educator. (Obtained from http://www.providentfoundation.org/history/pages/011.html)

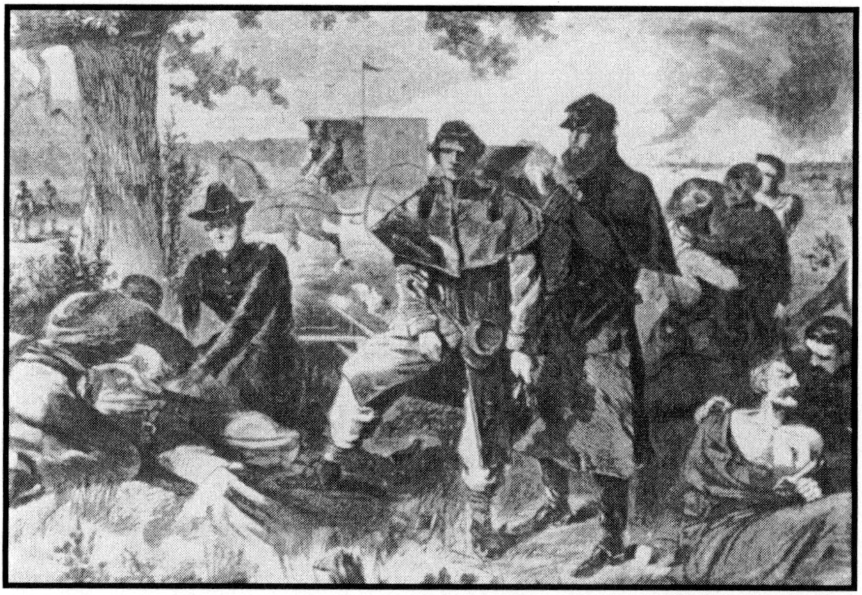

Figure 8. American Civil War (1861-1865) scene showing the treatment of a patient by a surgeon on the left side of the picture. (Wood engraving after Winslow Homer that appeared in Harper's Weekly, July 12, 1862; obtained from Lyons S and Petrucelly II RJ. *Medicine: An illustrated history*. New York: Harry N. Abrams Inc.; 1978)

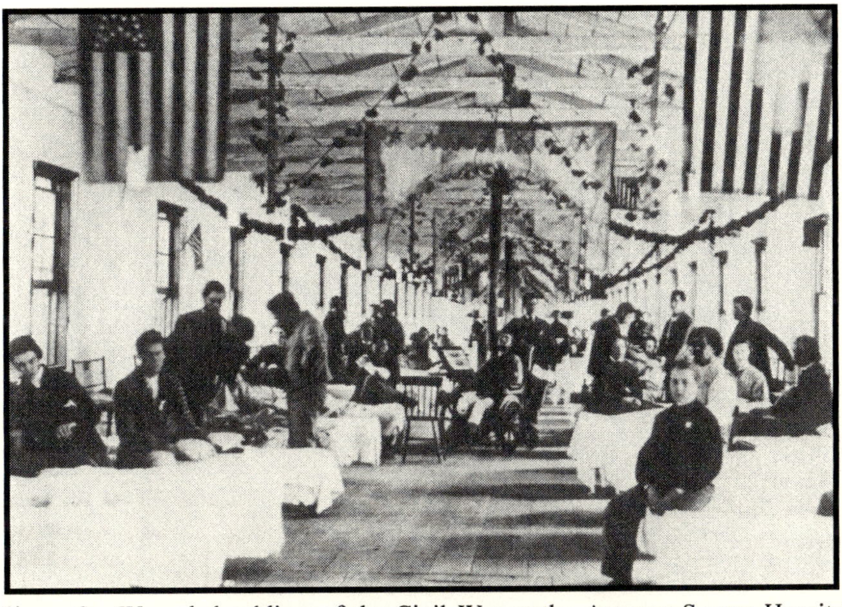

Figure 9. Wounded soldiers of the Civil War at the Armony Square Hospital. (Photograph by Matthew Brady, Harris Brisbane Dick Fund, Metropolitan Museum of Art, New York, obtained from Lyons S and Petrucelly II RJ. *Medicine: An illustrated history*. New York: Harry N. Abrams Inc.; 1978)

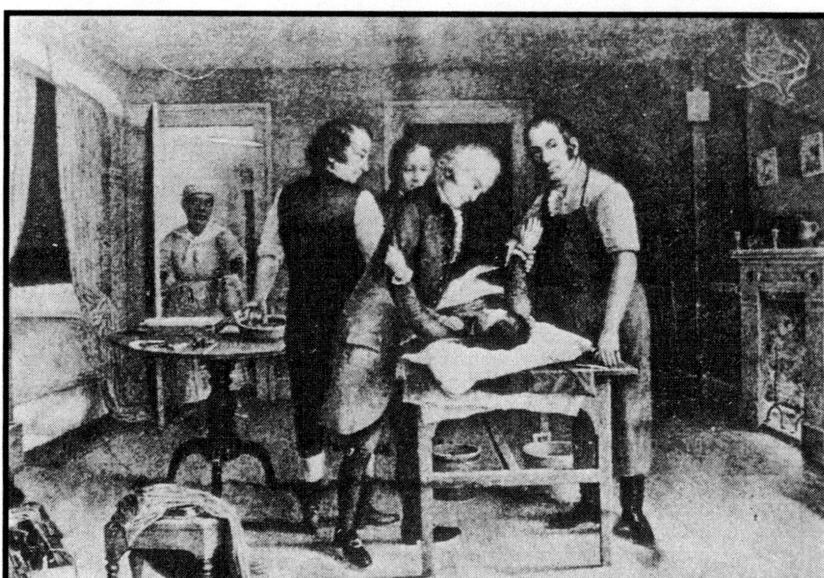

Figure 10. Ephraim McDowell (1771-1830) performing the first successful abdominal operation on the ovary of a cyst weighing several pounds in December 1809. (Reproduction of a sketch by Dr. Alban Goldsmith, Medical Communications Incorporated; obtained from Lyons S and Petrucelly II RJ. *Medicine: An illustrated history*. New York: Harry N. Abrams Inc.; 1978)

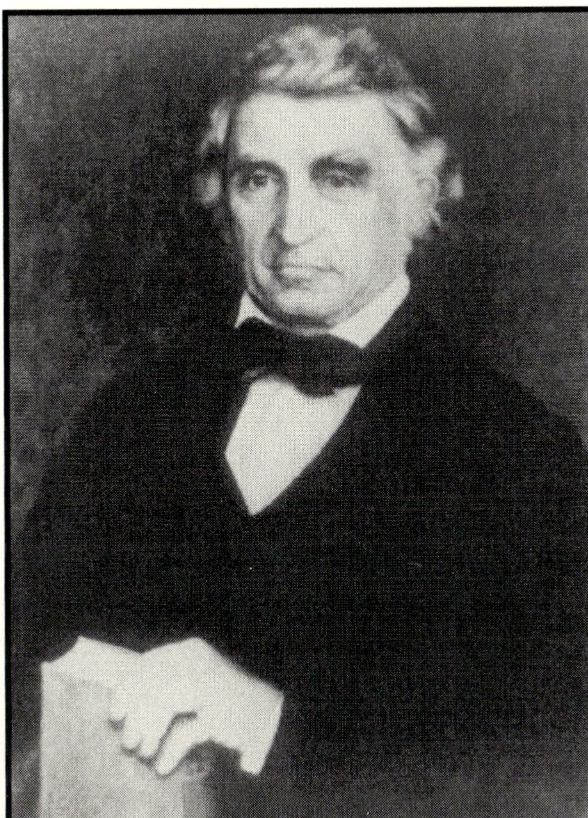

Figure 11. William Beaumont (1785-1853), noted military surgeon without formal training, made an incredible medical discovery on the decisive role of gastric juice in the physiology of digestion. He is considered to be the Father of Gastric Physiology. (Painting kept at National Library of Medicine, Bethesda, MD; obtained from Lyons S and Petrucelly II RJ. *Medicine: An illustrated history.* New York: Harry N. Abrams Inc.; 1978)

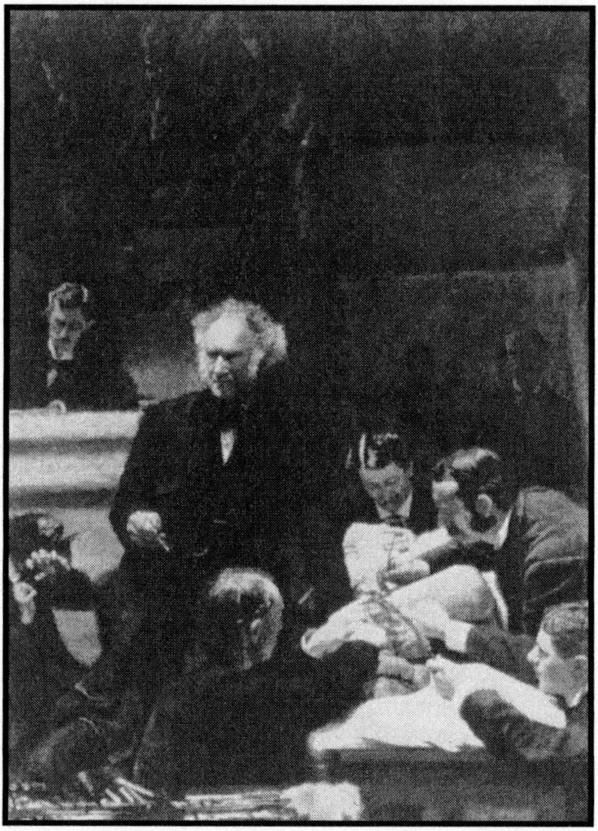

Figure 12. *The Gross Clinic*, a painting depicting Professor Samuel D. Gross performing a bone sequestrectomy for osteomyelitis in the lower extremity. Thomas Eakins created this magnificent work of art in 1875. (Jefferson Medical College, Thomas Jefferson University, Philadelphia, PA; obtained from Lyons S and Petrucelly II RJ. *Medicine: An illustrated history*. New York: Harry N. Abrams Inc.; 1978)

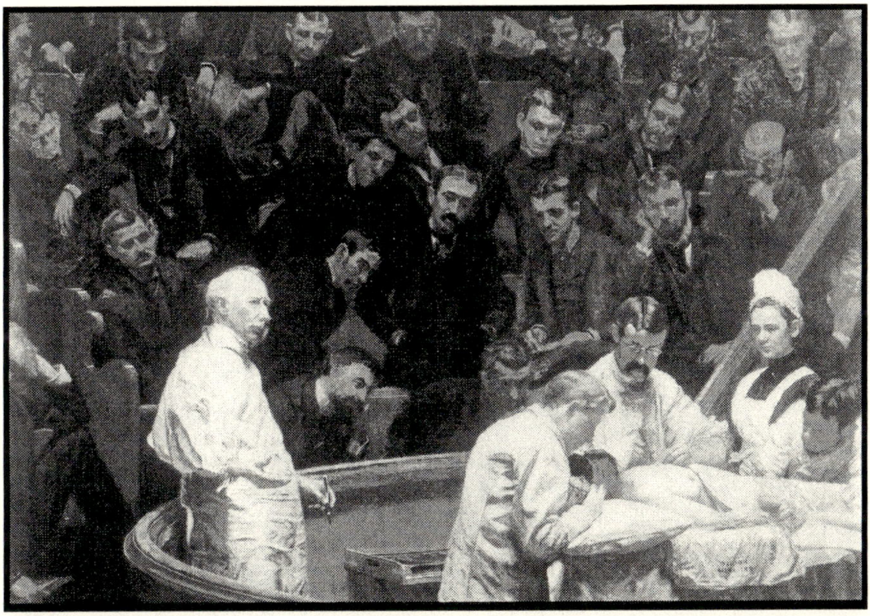

Figure 13. *The Agnew Clinic*, a painting depicting Professor Agnew performing breast surgery for cancer. Thomas Eakins took to the canvas this very unique work of art in 1889. (University of Pennsylvania School of Medicine, Philadelphia, PA; obtained from Lyons S and Petrucelly II RJ. *Medicine: An illustrated history*. New York: Harry N. Abrams Inc.; 1978)

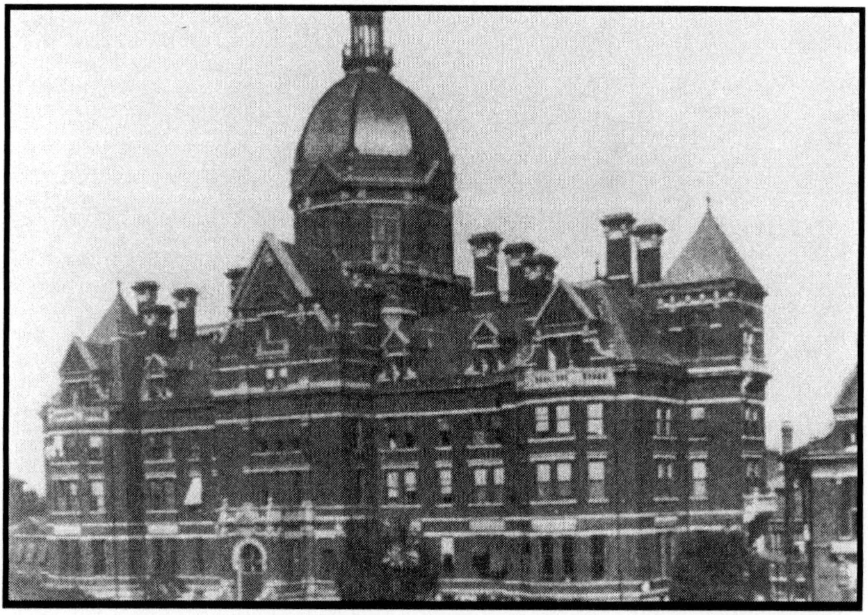

Figure 14. Photograph of the Johns Hopkins Hospital and School of Medicine (1893) designed by John Shaw Billings (1893-1913). This new institution took the lead in medicine in the United States. (The Alan Mason Chesney Medical Archives of the Johns Hopkins Medical Institutions, Baltimore, MD; obtained from Rutkow IM. *Surgery: AN Illustrated History*. St. Louis, MO: Mosby-Year Book Inc; 1993.)

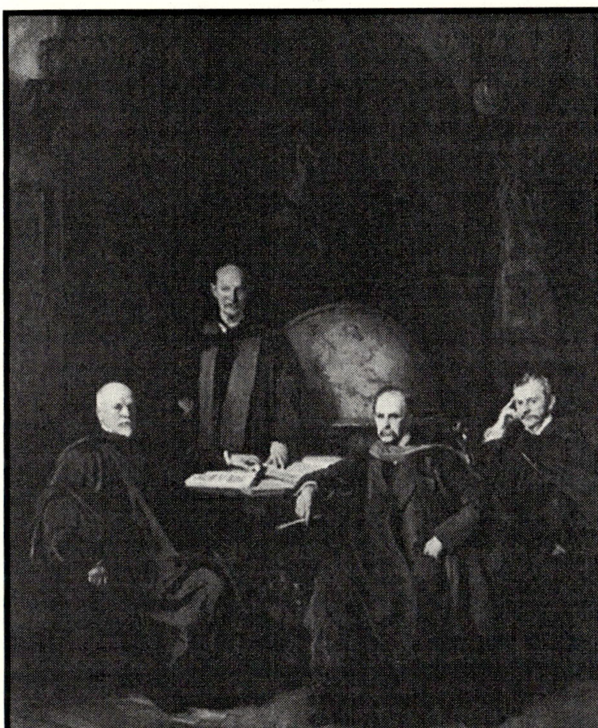

Figure 15. *The Four Doctors*, a panting representing the four physicians who founded Johns Hopkins Hospital and School of Medicine. John Singer Sargent (1856-1925) included, from left to right, Welch, Halsted, Osler, and Kelly as the basis of this extraordinary work of art (1906). (Johns Hopkins Medical Institutions, Baltimore, MD; obtained from http://en.wikipedia.org/wiki/William_Osler.)

CHAPTER 7
NOT FOR WHITE MEN ONLY

Up to the first third of the nineteenth century, American medicine was not an exception to that of other countries where women and minorities were not accepted within the mainstream of medical practice. In the late eighteenth century, the newly founded medical schools in the United States of America did not have provisions for considering women with the entering classes of medical students. At the same time, black Americans were at a level equal to or even worse than that of women since slavery had not yet been eliminated. In this writing, we analyze the incorporation of women and African Americans into the ranks of the American medical profession.

Women in American Medicine

General Aspects

American doctors were reluctant to accept women in organized medicine even up to the time of the Civil War. The reasons were not clear, but traditionalism, Victorian values, impulsive and irrational female behavior, passivity of mind, and weakness of body were all cited as important detractors for women to be considered as potential doctors. However, no substantive evidence was offered as a good reason to prevent the education of female physicians. Regina Markell Morantz, dedicated student of women doctors of the nineteenth century, presented the following rationale utilized by physicians during the second half of that century: "While denying them (females) access to the kind of education they could approve, critics held their alleged inferior training against them, often refusing to consult with women physicians and ostracizing male practitioners who did" (*The Connecting Link*, p. 163).

Women who wanted to be physicians ignored negative reasoning and moved ahead with their desire to reach their goals. However hard it was, they persevered in their professional inclination. Women's motivations varied from wishing to make a living to opportunities for knowledge in science. They prepared themselves well to establish good communication with the reluctant orthodox medical establishment. The break came in 1847 when the first woman was accepted in an American medical school.

Elizabeth Blackwell (1821-1910)

Elizabeth Blackwell (Figure 6) was the first woman to obtain a medical degree (MD) in the United States in 1849, from Geneva Medical College in upstate New York. She moved from England with her family in 1832 and had to combat rejection and continuous criticism to reach her main objective of becoming an MD, a long and arduous road! Blackwell had prepared herself very well by the time she applied to medical school, but this did not convince medical school authorities that she was a good candidate. When she finally was accepted by Geneva Medical College, according to Kent, it was due to the fact that the students decided to play a joke on the dean who stated to them that if all agreed she would be accepted in the school. The prospect of admitting a woman was so inconceivable that the dean never thought they would agree. To oppose him, all students answered affirmatively, and thus the first woman was accepted to medical school. As time went by, she turned out to be an asset to the school but not enough to convince the administration that females should be routinely considered for admission in subsequent years. Although none were accepted thereafter, Geneva's only shield from historical obscurity was its one and only woman student.

One long fight had been won by Blackwell, but the battle continued. When she finished her academic work and began applying for a hospital position to achieve her clinical experience, rejections poured again. Because of this, she decided to leave the United States and to travel to France where she found a position at *La Maternité Hospital* in Paris. Dedication and hard work were the norm for her. Unfortunately, while in this position, she contracted a severe infection in the left eye that required removal of the eye and the need to wear an artificial replacement.

After less than a year in France, Blackwell moved to London, England, where she continued her training at St. Bartholomew's Hospital. She had the support of the eminent surgeon Sir James Paget while in England and in 1851 returned to New York City to start her medical practice in America. Since she had few patients because of the stigma of being a woman doctor, she dedicated herself to teaching medical and sex education, became involved in social causes, and developed a hospital and a new medical school. She believed,

> that male doctors did not understand a woman's needs and that many women were afraid to go to a man for medical help. She dreamed of starting a hospital for female patients run by women doctors (Kent, 19).

In 1857, Elizabeth and Emily Blackwell (a younger sister who also had graduated from an American medical school) and Dr. Marie Zakrzewska founded the New York Infirmary for Women and Children. Ten years later, in 1868, the Blackwells founded the Women's Medical College of the New York Infirmary. The school remained under the care of Emily, and Elizabeth returned to England in 1869 where she lived and worked until her death.

In 1874, Blackwell helped to establish the London School of Medicine for Women. She continued to teach her favorite topics of women's health, sex education, hygiene, and the moral education of children. She wrote extensively and introduced the importance of seeing patients as whole persons where the spirit was comforted as much as the body. Blackwell retired from the practice of medicine at the age of 73, in 1894. Thirteen years later, she left teaching all together. On May 31, 1910, at the age of 89, she died in Hastings, England.

It is not hard to accept that the medical profession is better due to the extraordinary pioneering steps taken by Elizabeth Blackwell (Figure 6). According to Kent, at the time of her death, 7,399 women were licensed physicians and surgeons in the United States. This was an incredible realization of the power of her will and her determination in pursuing with dedicated vigor an important and single cause: the opportunity for women to be considered candidates to become doctors in equal standing with men.

First Medical Schools to Accept Women in the United States

In 1847, Geneva Medical College in upstate New York became the first school to accept women in the United States. In 1849, after Elizabeth Blackwell graduated, school officials reversed their position and did not consider women for acceptance. Two years later, the Eclectic Central Medical College in Syracuse began accepting women and thus, it should be considered the first truly coeducational medical school in the country. In 1850, the Woman's (initially Female) Medical College of Pennsylvania was created by the Quakers as an important example of single-sex medical education in the United States and the world. A few years later, the Cleveland Medical College started to accept women. Marie Zakrzewska and Emily Blackwell were among their prominent graduates.

In 1856, the New England Female Medical College received a charter from the state of Massachusetts to incorporate their activities within the law. In this school, Dr. Marie Zakrzewka took a prominent role as a teacher. In 1862, she founded the New England Hospital of Boston with the purpose of providing women with medical care by physicians of the same sex. In 1863, the Homeopathic New York Medical College for Women in New York City was established. Clemence Lozier, an early medical school graduate, played an important position in raising the number of female students accepted at this college. In 1868, the Blackwells, Elizabeth and Emily, established the Women's Medical College of the New York Infirmary. By 1870, some of the leading orthodox mainstream medical schools began considering the acceptance of women in their medical classes. In this category was the respected University of Michigan Medical School which became coeducational in that year.

As the nineteenth century advanced, women were more recognized as potential physicians in the medical arena. By 1882, 17 state medical societies opened their doors to women. In 1884, the Massachusetts Medical Society approved the acceptance of women as members. By 1893, women were considered for matriculation at Tufts University Medical School, Boston University, and Johns Hopkins Medical School, which had opened its doors that year. Cornell Medical School followed suit in 1899. It appeared, then, that women were making real progress in claiming their rights.

Some Other Notable Women Physicians in the United States

Elizabeth Blackwell was not the only prominent woman physician of her generation. Other distinguished women helped to promote the cause of education and equal rights for women in medicine. Some of these women accomplished a great deal! Brief statements of the first female physicians of the nation will be presented below.

Lydia Folger Fowler (1822-1879)

Lydia Folger Fowler became the first American-born woman doctor when she graduated from the Central Medical College of Syracuse in 1850 and the second woman to receive a medical degree in the United States. The first had been Elizabeth Blackwell, born in England, who received her MD in 1849. For a short period of time, in 1851, the Rochester Eclectic Medical College recruited Fowler to become a professor of midwifery and diseases of women and children, becoming in this way the first female professor at an American medical school. It was a short-lived stint since the school closed a year later.

As with many women physicians of the time, Fowler had to overcome the difficulty in having a regular medical practice which could sustain itself especially since sectarian and irregular medicine was still abundant in the 1860s. She surmised that it would be better to concentrate on health education and disease prevention than on other aspects of medical care. In 1860, she went to England and France to study for a year and then returned to the United States. A year later, in 1862, she returned to London where she remained until her death in 1879.

Emily Blackwell (1826-1910)

Another distinguished member of the Blackwell clan was Emily. Like her sister Elizabeth, Emily was born near Bristol, England. The Blackwell family moved to the United States when the father's refinery burned to the ground. In the new country and in due time, Emily followed in the footsteps of her sister Elizabeth. She immediately realized that in spite of her sister's encouragement, the road to medicine was filled with antagonism and road blocks throughout the entire journey. After multiple rejections and serious challenges, she graduated from Cleveland Medical College (today Case Western Reserve) in 1854, five years after her sister Elizabeth completed her studies at Geneva, New York.

After graduation, she pursued post-graduate clinical work in Britain, France, and Germany. Blackwell went first to work with the prominent obstetrician/gynecologist Sir James Young Simpson in Edinburgh, Scotland. Simpson had innovative ideas as to how to produce anesthesia with chloroform during surgical procedures including the birth of a child of Queen Victoria. Blackwell then moved to the Children's Hospital in London to work under the tutelage of Dr. William Jenner—no relation to Edward Jenner, pioneer of smallpox vaccination—who was a leader in the study of infectious diseases. From here, Blackwell proceeded to the surgical and medical clinics of Paris, Berlin, and Dresden. She thus completed excellent surgical and medical studies for two years before returning to the United States.

Once in this country, Blackwell concentrated on developing and supporting the New York Infirmary for Women and Children which was founded in 1857. In this hospital, she remained as chief of surgery and helped with other matters. In 1868, she founded a medical school with Elizabeth that remained open until 1898 when it merged with Cornell. In 1900, Blackwell retired from practice, and ten years later she passed away on September 7, 1910.

Marie Elizabeth Zakrzewska (1829-1902)

Of German and Polish descent, Marie Zakrzewska graduated from midwifery school in 1851 in Berlin. Her teacher and supporter, Dr. Joseph Schmidt, died a year later and left Zarkzewska unprotected in a medical world dominated by men. In 1853, she came to the United States with a younger sister. With the help of Elizabeth Blackwell, Zakrzewska attended Cleveland Medical College in the Midwest and graduated in 1856 with an MD. Immediately thereafter, she moved east to New York where she helped the Blackwell sisters develop and establish the New York Infirmary for Women and Children in 1857. Elizabeth was the physician in charge while Emily Blackwell was the dedicated surgeon and Zakrzewska the obstetrician and general manager.

In 1859, Zakrzewska moved to Boston to become professor of obstetrics and diseases of women and children at the New England Female Medical College. Unfortunately, things did not work out since the owner of the school, Samuel Gregory, shared few of Zakrzewska's views on medical education. Three years later, she resigned and founded the New England Hospital for Women and Children in Boston. She dedicated the rest of her life to enhancing the opportunities for young women to be effectively educated in the field of medicine. "Dr. Zak (as many affectionately called her) was the greatest force in insuring the early success of women doctors in America" (Stille, p. 79). She retired in 1899 and three years later died of a stroke. She left a significant void in the support of the causes to improve women's medical education and training.

Other Notable American Women Physicians

Many other courageous American women delved into the field of medicine. Chronologically, we encounter Sarah Parker Redmond (1826-1894), Black American physician and activist who finished her medical studies at Santa Maria Nuova Hospital in Florence, Italy, in 1868, but did not receive her formal graduation papers at the time. Rebecca Lee was the first Black American physician; she graduated from the New England Female Medical College in Boston in 1864 and practiced in Virginia. Rebecca J. Cole (1848-1922) was the first Black woman to graduate from the Women's Medical College of Pennsylvania in 1867 and practiced medicine in New York, North Carolina, Washington, D.C., and Philadelphia.

Emily Horton Cleveland (1829-1878) graduated from the Female Medical College in 1855, where she gave her services for some time. In 1862, she took the position of chief resident at the Woman's Hospital of Philadelphia. She continued to work at this institution until her death. Mary Harris Thompson (1829-1895) completed her studies at the New England Female Medical College in 1863, and then moved to Chicago where she founded the Women's Hospital Medical College in 1870. She pursued her medical education work and practice in Chicago where she passed away. Mary Edwards Walker (1832-1919) graduated from Syracuse Medical College in 1853. She became the first woman U.S. army surgeon. In 1865, she was given the Congressional Medal of Honor for Meritorious Service, which Congress took away in 1917 because of her supposed lack of merit. Her eccentric views and unique wardrobe did not help the case of this very controversial woman physician.

A great number of distinguished medical women followed in the steps of their predecessors. In this book, we have limited our writing to cover only the group mentioned above because of the scope of our work. As the twentieth century advanced, medical education of women became part of the mainstream, and women were not excluded from the decision making any longer.

Blacks in American Medicine

General Aspects

African Americans did not receive a meaningful opportunity to participate in the national medical scene until decades after the Civil War was won. Once the

North and South settled their differences over the issue of slavery and Robert E. Lee surrendered to Ulysses S. Grant on April 9, 1865, the nation began the much awaited period of reconstruction. The 13th Amendment of the Constitution (1865) legally eliminated slavery throughout the country. The social reality was different since most of the southern states continued the same social order of white supremacy. In many ways, this environment affected the slow incorporation of blacks into American medicine.

In spite of a difficult national climate for the acceptance of blacks into active society, including the medical world, changes began to occur in the medical education scene. A few years after the Civil War, in 1869, Howard University School of Medicine, an eminent predominantly black school, was established in Washington, D.C., by General O. O. Howard, director of the Freedman's Bureau. Several years later, in 1876, Meharry Medical College, an exclusively black college, opened its doors in Nashville.

Evolution continued on its way but needed the active disposition of blacks to claim their rights, and it did occur in that way. Black physicians organized their own hospitals and medical societies. In fact, the national black organization for physicians, the National Medical Association, was established in 1895 because the American Medical Association had negative policies for admitting blacks into the organization.

First Black American Physicians

Although there were many black individuals involved in medicine at the beginning of the colonies and thereafter, the most prominent was Lucas Santomée Peters who Robert C. Hayden, well-known black American historian, described in the following manner:

> As early as 1667, an African by the name of Lucas Santomée Peters was trained in medicine in Holland. He practiced in the colony of New York under the Dutch and the British. When the British took over New York, the governor gave him land in return for medical services (p. 11).

Other black slaves learned from their masters the medicine of the day such as Primus and Papan who took over the medical practices of their masters after they passed away. Their medical treatments were appreciated by their loyal patients.

Three physicians have been extensively recognized as black pioneers in the practice of medicine in the country. James Derham, born a slave in 1757 in

Philadelphia, served under doctors John Kearsley, a Dr. West (no first name identified), and Robert Love until he obtained his freedom and opened a medical practice in New Orleans in 1783. Dr. Benjamin Rush, father of American medicine, recognized his ability and invited him to return to Philadelphia, which he did. Derham was recognized and admired by the medical profession, particularly in throat disorders and diseases associated with climate changes. Rush, the great American master, said of Derham:

> I have conversed with him upon most of the most acute and epidemic diseases of the country where he lives and was pleased to find him perfectly acquainted with the modern simple mode of practice on these diseases. I expected to have to suggest some new medicines to him but he suggested many more to me (ohoh.essortment.com/africanamerican_rqdo.htm, p. 1)

James McCune Smith (1813-1865) was the second of this triumvirate of black American physician pioneers. He distinguished himself from an early age as a brilliant young man. Peter Williams, an Episcopalian priest, helped him to enroll at the University of Glasgow in Scotland at age 19. There he obtained a BA in 1835, an MA a year later, and an MD in 1837. In the farewell dinner given to him by his friends in Scotland, he was praised for all of his accomplishments, and he took to the floor to state:

> 'I thank you for the sake of my countrymen—that part of them, especially, who participate in such an unholy prejudice—for it must prove to them that you, who also have a complexion as fair, if not fairer than their own—that you are not only free from such prejudice, but glory in being free from it. Awaiting me will be insults which harm not the body but which enter the soul. The memory of this evening will cheer me on to endure the oppressor's scorn.' He concluded by pledging that it [would] be his life-long struggle to participate in the downfall of slavery and uplift of the free people of color in America (ohoh.essortment.com/africanamerican_rqdo.htm, p. 2).

Upon his return to his native country, he established a very successful medical practice and was considered one of the best physicians of the new country.

David J. Peck was the third physician of this notable group. From 1844 to 1846, he was apprenticed to Dr. Joseph P. Gazzen. Immediately thereafter, he entered Rush Medical College in the fall of 1846 and graduated a year later. He became the first black physician to graduate from an American medical school. He practiced medicine in Philadelphia from 1849 to 1851 after touring the state of

Ohio with William Lloyd Garrison and Frederick Douglass following his graduation from Rush. At the insistence of his childhood friend, Martin Delany, Peck joined him to found a home for free blacks in Central America. He remained in this land until at least 1855, after which time there are no records of his whereabouts.

Another distinguished black American physician was Martin R. Delany. He was a free black who was born in 1812 in Charleston, West Virginia, and grew up in Pennsylvania. He began his medical apprenticeship in Pittsburgh at the age of 19. Delany dedicated himself to freeing slaves for a while and in 1851 returned to Pittsburgh to continue his medical studies. He was not accepted at the University of Pennsylvania and several schools in New York because of his race. Finally, Harvard Medical School admitted him. After attending classes for a year, he traveled the country defending the intelligence of black Americans. Delany returned to Pittsburgh to practice medicine and in 1854 was a leader in treating patients with cholera during that year's epidemic. He participated in the city board and later served during the Civil War as a major in the Union Army. As was the custom for black physicians of the time, he dedicated a great deal of his effort to improving the education and conditions of black Americans. He is acknowledged as one of the earliest black nationalists and African American politicians in the United States.

Many more black physicians were important in the United States, and therefore, it would be hard to be totally comprehensive. These are some names that Herbert M. Morais, noted scholar of black history, referred to in his important treatise on *The History of the Negro in Medicine*. He presented those that were self-taught healers in the early nineteenth century such as James Still, David Ruggles, and Martin Wells Brown. Thereafter, he introduced trained physicians who were the rule in the middle of the same century. In this case, he described Charles Dunbar, Daniel Laing Jr., Isaac Humphrey Snowden, John S. Rock, Major Alexander T. Augusta, and John V. DeGrasse.

Other Prominent Black American Physicians

Dale Hale Williams (1856-1931) (Figure 7) was born in Hollidaysburg, Pennsylvania, but roamed around various places after the death of his father because of his family's difficult economic conditions. After moving to near Janesville, Wisconsin, he became an apprentice to Dr. Henry Palmer in 1878.

Two years later, he entered Northwestern University Medical School. He graduated in 1883 and opened his medical office in Chicago, Illinois. Williams attended patients and operated on them, using the most up-to-date advances of the day. He was appointed surgeon of the South Side Dispensary in Chicago and clinical instructor in anatomy at Northwestern. In 1891, he established the Provident Hospital, which demonstrated an extraordinary overall success rate of 87%, very unique results for the conditions of the time. On July 9, 1893, he made history by operating upon a young black man, James Cornish, with a stab injury to the chest. He opened the chest, noted bleeding in the pericardium, and sutured it. Fifty-one days later, Cornish left Provident Hospital in excellent health. This surgery was noteworthy in that Dr. Williams opened the chest cavity with success which was considered a daring advance of the day.

In 1894, Daniel Williams moved to Washington, D.C., where he became chief surgeon at the Freedmen's Hospital. In this institution, he reorganized all medical and surgical practices, developed pathological and bacteriological units, recruited highly qualified doctors, and began an internship program. Physicians started to recognize Williams abilities and organizational skills. Frequent visits by other physicians became part of the Freedmen's routine. On another front, Williams was a founding member of the National Medical Association and the American College of Surgeons. He was also a member of the Chicago Surgical Society. He left a unique imprint on the medicine of this country and the world.

Several other black American physicians were important contributors to medicine of the late nineteenth and early twentieth centuries in this country. George Cleveland Hall, Austin Maurice Curtis, Nathan Francis Mossell (born in 36Canada and educated in the United States), Henry R. Butler, Cornelius N. Dorsette, John A. Kenney, and A. M. Townesend were a few of the prominent black physicians of the time.

Solomon Carter Fuller (1872-1953) came to this nation from Monrovia, Liberia, in 1889. He attended Livingston College in North Carolina and graduated four years later. From there, he directed his efforts to graduating from Boston University School of Medicine in 1897. Upon graduation, Fuller continued his career at Westborough State Hospital for the Insane in Massachusetts. In this institution as well as at Boston University School of Medicine, Fuller committed his entire professional life—until 1933 when he retired—to the study of neurological diseases. His contributions were many in scientific matters in addition to his enormous impact on the education of black American physicians. He was a counselor and friend to a large number of people and lived a long, meaningful, and engaged life.

As time went by, black American physicians increased their presence and contributions to this country. Hayden, in his well-researched book, *11 African American Doctors*, reviewed the life and accomplishments of eleven black American doctors. In it, he demonstrated the character and significance of their lives. Because the scope of this book does not extend beyond the first third of the twentieth century, we have presented only two of those great black American physician pioneers, Daniel Williams and Solomon Fuller. The other nine doctors (William A. Hinton, Louis T. Wright, William Montague Cobb, Arthur C. Logan, Daniel A. Collins (a dentist researcher), Jane C. Wright, Eugene W. Adams (a veterinarian), Angela D. Ferguson, and Charles R. Drew) of which seven were physicians, are not included in this writing because their work occurred beyond the 1930s. Their names, however, should serve as an example for future generations of American physicians.

Howard, Meharry, and Others

Howard and Meharry represented the pillars of medical education for blacks in the United States. Both colleges were founded as an essential place for blacks to be educated in medical affairs and accepted women from the outset. Both schools were chartered after the Civil War with ten years' difference. Howard was biracial, and Meharry accepted blacks exclusively. James L. N. Bowen and George W. Brooks were the first black physicians to be graduated from Howard Medical School in 1871. The first woman graduate was Mary Dora Spackman in 1872. James Monroe Jamison was the first black student to obtain an MD from Meharry Medical College in 1877.

Todd Savitt, noted medical historian and student of black medical education, recently reviewed all black medical colleges established in the United States from 1868 to 1920 (1985b). There were 14 black medical colleges founded in that period of time. Only two of this group remained open, Howard and Meharry. The other twelve colleges closed between four and thirty-six years after their founding. This account offers a good perspective of the incredible feat realized by those colleges that remain active even up to the present time.

Howard and Meharry were able to battle many difficult financial times by the endurance of the faculty's commitment to advancing medical education among black American citizens. They both represented a clear example of dedication and perseverance in maintaining and improving black medical education.

A Few Other Remarks

The antagonistic forces evident in white America that prevented blacks from obtaining satisfactory medical education remained alive long after the Civil War, long after the introduction of constitutional amendments to incorporate blacks as full-fledged citizens, and long after the beginning of the twentieth century. The period of progress was prolonged and arduous. It would take many years until after Martin Luther King, Jr.'s march in 1963 that racial equality would become a high priority in the country's agenda. In 1967, President Johnson called for a commission to review the status of black rights in the country. Governor Otto Kerner of Illinois, chairman of the commission, reported in March 1968, that significant changes were needed to overcome the great inequalities existing in black America. The conditions of black American medical education were not quite as grim, but suffered a slow and incomplete restoration.

By the 1970s, practically all medical schools in the country were accepting competent black students, an extraordinary change compared to what was occurring in the first half of the century. It appeared, then, that African Americans in medicine were on a road of continuous and permanent improvement in professional opportunities.

Conclusion

Before 1849, there were no women with MDs obtained from any medical school in the United States. That year marked the first time in which a woman, Elizabeth Blackwell, received an MD from an American school, Geneva Medical College in upstate New York. Despite this milestone, women continued to be rejected from the practicing medical schools in the country. Persistence and determination from those women wanting to be doctors created the necessary movement to develop all-female medical schools and hospitals and generated enough pressure on the standard leading medical schools of the day.

In 1870, the University of Michigan Medical School became coeducational. By 1882, there were 115 female members of 17 state medical societies. In 1893, Johns Hopkins University School of Medicine received half a million dollars from women's generous gifts, particularly Mary Garrett, with the understanding that female students would be admitted under the same conditions as men. Immediately thereafter, a slew of exclusively male medical schools opened their doors to competent women desirous of being doctors. The tide had been turned!

Black American medical education, for different reasons, followed a similar pattern. Black Americans were not accepted in American medicals schools until 1846 when David Peck graduated from Rush Medical College in Chicago in 1847. James Derham, an apprentice-trained physician, practiced medicine in New Orleans and his native Philadelphia beginning in 1783. Other distinguished black American physicians such as James McCune Smith and Martin R. Delany practiced medicine in the mid-nineteenth century as well. Acceptance of blacks in traditionally white dominant medical schools was a rare phenomenon. It took the American Civil War and more until isolated consideration was given to some black American students. Because of the discriminating status of the American medical profession in general, black colleges and universities were developed. Howard University, in 1868, showed the way by founding its own medical school. Meharry Medical College followed suit, and in 1876 founded their school. In 1895, the National Medical Association for black physicians was established as a response to the black non-inclusive policy of the American Medical Association.

The twentieth century was not an easy road for black Americans wanting to enter medicine. By the first third of the century, Howard and Meharry were producing the majority of black physicians in the country. The Civil Rights Movement did not appear to have a direct effect in significantly increasing the number of black doctors graduating from traditionally white medical schools. It was not until the second half of the twentieth century, particularly after 1970, that black Americans began to be considered in a more consistent fashion within the regular admission process of the majority of medical schools.

CHAPTER 8
NATION UP IN ARMS*

The American Civil War (1861-1865) introduced an extraordinary opportunity for the practice of medicine in the areas of wound management, care of the injured, and transportation of the sick. The war provided a large and comprehensive laboratory with all kinds of patients. The difficulty resided in finding an effective therapy for all types of problems, especially those associated with overcrowding maladies such as the large number of infectious diseases present at the time. Twice as many soldiers died from sickness and disease than from battlefield injuries

This section reviews the medical history of the Civil War from the medical statistics accumulated, the care of the injured and diseased soldiers, the competency of the medical practitioners, the development of the Sanitary Commission, and the medical advances introduced throughout the whole episode.

Medical Statistics

More than one million Americans soldiers fought against each other during the Civil War. The total number of deaths in the war was 624,571. Table 8.1 indicates the number of dead and wounded on both sides as well as the total number of losses.

Table 8.1. Casualties During American Civil War

	Dead	Wounded	Total Casualties
Union	364,511	281,881	646,392
Confederate	260,000	194,000	454,000
Total	624,511	485,881	1,100,392

From ehistory.com.uscw

* Partially published in *J Invest Surg*, 17:115-117 and 17:185-189, 2004, by Toledo-Pereyra LH and Toledo AH.

The Civil War took more Americans than any other war in the history of the country (Table 8.2). Until the Vietnam War, the fatal casualties observed in all other American wars combined were not as extensive as the ones seen in the Civil War. The magnitude of this event in the history of the nation cannot be overstated. Death ran rampant in the fields of this war. The Civil War took place before the availability of advanced and sophisticated treatments in the management of regular diseases and injuries received on the battlefield (Table 8.3).

Table 8.2. Fatal Casualties of the American Wars

Event	Total Number of Deaths (soldiers)
Revolutionary War	4,435
War of 1812	2,260
Mexican War	13,283
Spanish-American War	2,246
World War I	116,516
World War II	405,399
Korean War	33,746
Vietnam War	58,152
Civil War	624,511

From ehistory.com.uscw

For four years, Americans grew accustomed to the devastating effects of a war fought among brothers, friends, and neighbors. Thousands of lives could not be spared in this gruesome and horrendous spectacle.

Table 8.3. Estimated Civil War Deaths Due to Battle or Infection and/or Disease

	Number of Deaths	
Cause of Death	Union	Confederate
Battle	110,000	95,000
Infection and/or Disease	250,000	165,000

From ehistory.com.uscw

Fevers, intestinal diseases, and pulmonary diseases were among the causes of death during the Civil War (Table 8.4). Confederates experienced a higher percentage of these causes of death. The Union Army overall had a higher number of deaths due to battle.

Table 8.5 covers the top ten battles based on casualties fought in the Civil

War. It reviews the number of forces engaged, the military commanders, and the ultimate outcome of the battles. When one examines who, whether the Union or the Confederacy, won more battles in these main events, no clear winner emerges from these hard fought encounters. It is debatable whether the nation as a whole reached improved economical, social, and political status because of it. The impact of the Civil War on medicine of the time and immediately thereafter will be addressed in this section.

Table 8.4. Other Important Medical Statistics from the U.S. Civil War		
Cause of Death	Union (%)	Confederate (%)
Continued Fevers	22	33
Malarial Fevers	0.9	1.1
Eruptive Diseases	5.3	5.1
Intestinal Diseases	1.2	1.4
Pulmonary Diseases	2.3	19
For Union Army: 1 in 4 chance of dying, 1 in 5 died from wounds, 1 in 13 died of disease, 1 in 10 wounded in action, 1 in 15 captured or reported missing, 1 in 7 captured died in prison.		

From ehistory.com.uscw

Care of the Injured and Diseased Soldiers

The number of physicians available at the start of the war was incredibly low, and they were ill prepared to undertake the care of the unexpectedly high number of injured and diseased soldiers. There was not enough time or adequate institutions that could train the medical staff who were planning to deliver care to wounded or diseased soldiers. The Union Army medical staff consisted of a surgeon general, thirty surgeons, and eighty-three assistant surgeons when the war began. Of these, twenty-four resigned to help the Confederacy and three other assistant surgeons were declared disloyal, an incredible state of affairs for a war that would carry such a disproportionately high mortality and morbidity all throughout its initial battles.

The Confederate Army medical staff was as ineffective as the Union side. In fact, because the Confederate medical staff needed to be created from the beginning, it was less organized and equipped than the Union counterpart. The Confederates depended on the will of the state governors to recruit the surgeons and assistant surgeons needed for the care of the injured and diseased soldiers.

Table 8.5. Ten Most Important Battles Based on Casualties During the Civil War*

		Forces Engaged			Casualties		
Battle	Date(s)	CSA	USA	Winner	Overall	CSA	USA
Gettysburg	Jul. 1-3, 1863	75,000	82,289	Federals	51,112	28,063	23,049
Chickamauga	Sept. 19-20, 1863	66,326	58,222	Confederacy	34,624	18,454	16,170
Chancellorsville	May 1-4, 1863	60,892	133,868	Confederacy	30,099	12,821	17,278
Spotsylvania	May 8-19, 1864	50,000	83,000	Confederacy	27,399	9,000	18,399
Antietam (Sharpsburg)	Sept. 17, 1862	51,844	75,316	Draw	26,134	13,724	12,410
The Wilderness	May 5-7, 1864	61,025	101,895	Inconclusive	25,416	7,750	17,666
Second Manasas (Second Bull Run)	Aug. 29-30, 1862	48,527	75,696	Confederacy	25,251	9,197	16,054
Stone's River (Murfreesboro)	Dec. 31, 1862-Jan. 3, 1863	37,739	41,400	Federals	24,645	11,739	12,906
Shiloh	Apr. 6-7, 1862	40,655	62,682	Federals	23,741	10,694	13,047
Fort Donelson	Feb. 13-16, 1862	21,000	27,000	Federals	19,455	16,623	2,832

*Based on total casualties—killed, wounded, captured, and missing
CSA = Confederate States of America

Adapted from http://www.ehistory.com/wscw/features/medicine/cwsurgeon/statistics.cfm

Sanitary conditions on the battlefield, in the operating theater, and in the temporary field hospitals were dismal. Surgeons operated in dirty coats; well-developed antiseptic procedures were not utilized; surgeons wore no hats, masks, or gloves; and instruments and dressings were not consistently cleaned. Surgeons and staff had no regard for the germ theory of disease at this point in time. The findings of Semmel Weis on the use of antiseptic techniques such as the use of chlorinated lime to rinse the physicians' hands prior to obstetrical delivery had not been instituted. The antiseptic techniques according to Lister had not yet been published. This would not happen until 1867, two years after the Civil War had finished.

Surgeons were eager to operate within the first twenty-four hours of injury before infection would set in. Infections were frequently secondary to *Staphylococcus aureus*. The most usual operation was amputation, either of the flap or circular type. At the end of the war, barely fifty percent of the surgeons preferred the flap operation. Surgeons with experience could amputate a limb in less than ten minutes. Most of the amputations were performed on the extremities (Table 8.6). Other injury sites such as the head, neck, chest, and abdomen had a bad prognosis with high mortality. The most common ammunition during the Civil War was the "dreadful" Minie ball. These bullets were extraordinarily damaging on impact and shattered any bone with which they came in contact. Soldiers with slight wounds as well as those who were mortally wounded had little impression on the practicing surgeons who dedicated themselves to attend those wounded soldiers with a plausible chance of remaining alive. Surgeons had to make decisions based on prognosis and possibility of success. These were the days of Civil War medicine (Figure 8).

Table 8.6. Mortality Rate Depending on Site of Amputation

Site	Number of Amputations	Mortality (%)
Hip Joint	66	83
Thigh	6,369	54
Knee Joint	195	58
Lower Leg	5,523	33
Ankle Joint	161	25
Foot or Toe	1,519	6
Shoulder Joint	866	2
Upper Arm	5,510	24
Elbow Joint	40	8
Forearm	1,716	14
Wrist Joint	69	10
Hands or Fingers	7,902	3
Total	29,981	26

From Bollet AJ. Civil War Surgery: All Those Amputations. *Resident & Staff Phys.* March 1999:85.

Four or five days after surgery, patients would commonly develop surgical fevers, for which there was no specific treatment. Their presence carried a high mortality (around 90% for pyemia, which means pus in the blood). The cause of these fevers was infectious and most likely *Streptococcus pyogenes* or *Staphylococcus aureus*. Antibiotics were not available and would not appear until three quarters of a century later. Several disinfectants were available such as iodine, carbolic acid, bichloride of mercury, sodium hypochlorite, and other agents. These agents were only used for the treatment of wounds with severe evidence of infection. The disinfectants were not utilized to prevent wound infections. The relationship between germs and wound infection was not recognized by the great majority of American surgeons of the time. The later acceptance of the germ theory of disease would be the pivotal event in making the germ-wound relationship better recognized.

A detailed description of the manner in which the surgeon took care of his battlefield cases is described at USCivilWar.Net:

> The field hospital was hell on earth. The surgeon would stand over the operating table for hours without a let up. Men screamed in delirium, calling for loved ones, while others lay pale and quiet with the effect of shock. Only the division's best surgeons did the operating and they were called 'operators.'...The surgeon would wash out the wound with a cloth (in the Southern Army sponges were long exhausted) and probe the wound with his finger (the finger being usually used), or a probe perhaps, looking for bits of cloth, bone, or the bullet. If the bone was broken or a major blood vessel torn, he would often decide on amputation. Later in the War, surgeons would sometimes experiment with resection, but far more common was amputation.

Anesthesia was almost universally utilized in all soldiers undergoing surgical procedures. Chloroform was the favorite anesthetic, used 75% of the time through the open drop technique, with a 0.4% mortality. Ether was unfavorable because of the possibility of explosion due to its flammability. In addition to the anesthetic agent, patients would receive various doses of whiskey, opiates, and possibly quinine. All these substances were complementary to the regular anesthetic administered.

From the words of an unknown student of Civil War affairs, we can summarize the actual operative procedure during the Civil War in the following manner:

> The surgeon usually had an operating table of a couple of boards between barrels. He usually had a rag soaked with chloroform, which was liberally doused. Today it is recognized as a dangerous

> procedure. Somehow, surgeons knew enough to periodically remove the rag or sponge. Therefore, few deaths resulted from chloroform poisoning. It is generally a myth that most operations were performed without anesthesia, with only a bullet to bite. Surgeons usually used the following procedure. First the surgeon would cut off the blood flow with a tourniquet. After that he would take a scalpel and slice through the outlying tissue and flesh. Then he would use a hacksaw-like tool called a capital saw to saw through the bone. It had replaceable blades. After the bone and flesh was sliced off, the surgeon would take silk sutures in the North and cotton sutures in the South, and sew the major arteries and veins together. The limb would be dropped on a pile that got thrown out after the day. Time was of the essence, so the soldier would be carried off of the platform and another soldier would be placed on the platform. This would take about fifteen minutes. (powerweb.net/bbock/war/amputate)

Patient care after the operative procedure was rudimentary. Hospitals were not all well supplied and personnel had no consistent techniques to follow. The care relied on the hands of assistant surgeons, nurses, and other medical personnel. There was no intravenous fluid administration; laboratory procedures to evaluate patients were non-existent; and radiological studies had not yet arrived. It took decades before each one of these therapeutic or diagnostic tests became available.

Competency of Medical Practitioners

The Civil War took place "at the end of the medical Middle Ages" (Civil War Medicine, ehistory.com). Science, technology, and medical care had not reached the desirable levels of success. There was practically no knowledge behind the treatments used during Civil War times. Surgical techniques varied a great deal, from primitive management to improved by still unacceptable modern treatments. Fallen soldiers had great chances of receiving poor care by an underprepared medical corps. As the war advanced in time, medical professionals and techniques simultaneously improved. By the end of the war, thousands of doctors, nurses, and volunteers had served during this glorious national nightmare (Figure 9).

At the time, the medical personnel of both Union and Confederate armies was highly unprepared and uneducated to deal with the health issues arising from the battlefield as well as the diseases affecting the general population.

The education of doctors during the Civil War was clearly insufficient.

Most of the physicians had served as apprentices instead of receiving formal training. Even those who attended medical school received poor training. In the United States, students of medicine spent less than two years in the classroom and no clinical experience or laboratory instruction was provided. Harvard Medical School "did not own a single stethoscope or microscope until after the war" (Civil War Medicine, ehistory.com). The education and training of other medical professionals such as assistant surgeons, nurses, and volunteers suffered from a similar lack of sophistication.

Table 8.7. Surgeon Generals and other Noted Military Medical Personalities Who Participated in the US Civil War	
Union	Confederacy
Surgeon Generals Dr. Thomas Lawson (1861) Dr. Clement Finlay (1861-1862) Dr. William Hammond (1862-1863) Dr. Joseph Barnes (1863-1865)	Surgeon Generals Dr. Samuel Preston Moore (1861-1865)
Other Medical Personalities Drs. Letterman, Smart, Woodward, Huntington, Otis, and others	Other Medical Personalities Drs. Stout, Madison, Haden, Langworthy, Potts, and others

The higher echelons of the medical departments of the Union and the Confederacy had, in general, competent physicians in charge of the operation. Some notable individuals were Dr. Samuel Preston Moore, surgeon general of the Confederacy, and Dr. Samuel Stout, superintendent of the Department of Tennessee. The Union had Dr. William Hammond as surgeon general and others including Drs. Joshua Letterman, Smart, Woodward, Huntington, and Otis. Many of these individuals represented the best that the nation could offer. Their participation was invaluable in accomplishing the goals set out at the beginning of the war. Table 8.7 lists the surgeon generals and other noted personalities that participated in the Civil War affairs.

Development of the United States Sanitary Commission

The United States Sanitary Commission was one of the great developments of the Civil War. The Sanitary Commission "was to do what the government could not do" (Civil War Medicine, ehistory.com). The Sanitary Commission grew from the important complementary support that women could offer to improve the care of the soldiers in the Civil War. The Sanitary

Commission, in spite of strong opposition by the War Department, President Lincoln, and the medical corps, was finally initiated on June 13, 1861, with the following purposes:

> To inquire into the recruiting service in the various States and by advice to bring them to a common standard; second, to inquire into the subjects of diet, clothing, cooks, camping grounds, in fact everything connected with the prevention of disease among volunteer soldiers not accustomed to the rigid regulations of regular troops; and third, to discover methods by which private and unofficial interest and money might supplement the appropriations of the Government. (civilwarhome.com/sanitarycommission)

The United States Sanitary Commission followed the steps of the British Sanitary Commission, which had helped in the Crimean War with functions that the government could not do. The Americans were organized under the leadership of two reformers, Dr. Elisha Harris, a noted public health figure, and the Reverend Henry Bellows, a distinguished Unitarian minister. But, in addition, the real support came from thousands of dedicated women, putting their efforts into building something that would duplicate and possibly improve upon the work of Florence Nightingale and her associates in the Crimean War. Frederick Law Olmsted, the outstanding New York landscape architect, was selected by Bellows to serve as the secretary of the commission, an important fit for this august body of sanitary reformers.

The commission remained occupied during most of the activities and battles of the Civil War. They sought, obtained, and brought needed supplies to the soldiers, improved nutrition, and they enhanced the sanitary program of the Union Army. The South did not have anything like it, and as a consequence they suffered. The principle of universality of relief established by the commission did not come through for the Confederacy; they had to rely on local or regional women's aid societies.

The commission organized branches in the various cities of the North which facilitated its function and ability to distribute all supplies and relief efforts to as many soldiers as possible. As the Civil War finished its hostilities, the commission did the same and closed its doors after having done an outstanding job in the care of the soldier on the government's side. Throughout its involvement during the Civil War, this generous and able group raised nearly twenty million dollars in money and supplies.

Other Important Highlights of the Civil War

We cannot finish this writing without emphasizing the role that "The Angels of the Battlefield" played in this most bloody contest. Nearly two thousand dedicated and unselfish women from both sides of the fight served as volunteer nurses in the hospitals of the Civil War. Dorothea Dix (1802-1887), at age 59, volunteered her services to the Union army. In June 1861, she became the Union's superintendent of Female Nurses. In this position, she organized an extraordinary army of volunteer Union nurses. She selected women who could perform the job effectively and who would be "plain looking and middle aged." Dix was stern, autocratic, self-reliant, highly committed, and dedicated to the nurses and soldiers' cause. She was an important contributor to the Union's goals. At war's end, she returned to her work on behalf of the mentally ill.

Another leader of great repute in the national goal to organize nurses during the Civil War was Clara Barton (1821-1912). She originated from Oxford, Massachusetts. In 1861, she was working for the U.S. Patent Office, outside of Washington, D.C., when she learned about the wounded who suffered from lack of medical supplies at the First Battle of Bull Run (Manassas). Due to this event, she joined the Union effort and organized an independent group to distribute medical supplies. She also served as superintendent of nurses in Major General Benjamin Butler's command, in addition to her nursing work at Virginia and South Carolina military hospitals. She continued her relief work after the war by contributing to the founding of the American Red Cross in 1881. Dix and Barton were clear and radiant pillars of the Union's nurse movement to improve medical care during the Civil War.

The Confederate side boasted some notable nurses as well. Sally Tompkins, Kate Cumming, Phoebe Pember, Ella Newsom, and other southern women were recognized leaders in the Confederate ranks. They all actively participated in caring for the sick and wounded, raising supplies for medical use, organizing funding events for financial support, and cooperating to plan strategic goals within the limitations of the Confederacy. Table 8.8 recognizes the important accomplishments of medical, nursing, and other key personnel during the American Civil War. Each one of the health components of the team provided a dedicated commitment to the goals of their particular group. The combined efforts resulted in better medical care.

Table 8.8. Important Accomplishments of Medical, Nursing, and Other Leaders During the Civil War

Leader	Side of Alliance	Accomplishments
Dr. William Hammond	Union	1. Introduced ridge ventilation. 2. Developed pavilion hospital design. 3. Introduced ambulance service. 4. Supported sanitary reforms. 5. Eliminated Calomel and Tartar emetic.* 6. Gave authority to medical directors.
Dr. Samuel P. Moore	Confederacy	1. Competitive exams for medical officers. 2. Better ventilation and cleaner hospitals. 3. Laboratories for drug manufacture, obtain medical supplies from Europe. 4. Distributed book on native southern herbs.
Dr. Jonathan Letterman	Union	1. Ambulance plan. 2. Organized medical supplies and care.
Nurses Dix and Barton (and other nurses)	Union	1. Developed nurses' volunteer program. 2. Enhanced care of patients. 3. Obtained supply for patients.
Henry Bellows and Frederick L. Olmsted (Sanitary Commission)	Union	1. Improved general sanitation. 2. Reached better nutrition. 3. Enhanced living conditions. 4. Better care for sick and injured.

*Calomel (mercurous chloride) was used for cleaning of bowels and as a general stimulant, and Tartar emetic was used for removal of poisons from stomach. Both were used excessively and caused intoxication. Therefore, Hammond banned them.

From ehistory.com.uscw and civilwarhome.com/medicine history

During the Civil War, a large number of natural medicines were utilized. Next, we introduce a brief description of the remedies recommended in those times:

> For rash they used red-oak bark and alum. Goose grease and sorghum, or honey, was a standard remedy for croup, backed up with turpentine and brown sugar. Sassafras tea was given in the spring and fall as a blood medicine. Adults' colds were doctored with horsemint tea and tea from the roots of broom sedge. For eruptions and impure blood, spice-wood tea was given. Wine was made from the berries of the elder bush. For diarrhoea, roots of blackberry and blackberry cordial; and so, also, was a tea made from the leaves of the rose geranium. Mutton suet, sweet gum and

> the buds of the balm of Gilead was a standard salve for all cuts and sores. Balsam cucumber was widely used as a tonic, and was considered a specific remedy in burns. Catnip, elecampane, and comfrey root and pennyroyal were in every good housewife's pantry, in which, also, was the indispensable string or red peppers, a bag of sage leaves and of 'balm.' Calamus root for colic in babies was a common dose. The best known standard Georgia tonic was dogwood, poplar and wild cherry barks, equal proportions, chipped fine and put in whiskey and taken wineglassfull at meal times; it is still used in large quantities from 'Yamacraw to Nickajack.' Dogwood, sumac and the roots of pine trees were largely used, and indigo was cultivated in the gardens. Instead of paregoric, fennel-seed tea was given to the babies. In hemorrhages, black haw root was commonly used. All the white mustard we had was raised in our gardens. (civilwarhome.com/drusshsp)

Druggists and physicians of the Civil War prescribed medicine substitutes for those products that needed to be imported from other places (Table 8.9). Imported medicines were hard to obtain and were at considerably higher prices. With limited supplies, not all of the medicines were readily available when required. Therefore, it was more practical to seek substitute medicines.

Table 8.9. Some Medical Compounds Recommended by Physicians and Druggists of the Civil War

Imported Articles	Substitutes
Columbo, Quassia	Yellow root, Spanish flies, potato bugs, powdered leaves of butternut
Jalap	Wild Jalap, Mulberry bark, Butternut, Dock, Wild potato vine, Amer Columbo
Quinine and Peruvian Bark	Tulip tree bark, Dogwood, Cotton-seed tea, Chestnut root and bark, Thoroughwort, Spanish oak bark, Knob grass, Willow bark
Digitalis	Blood-root, Wild cherry, Pipsissiwa, Bugle weed, Jasmine
Conium	American hemlock
Opium	American hemlock, Motherwort
Sarsaparilla	Wild Sarsaparilla, Soapwort, Yellow parilla, China briar, Queen's delight
Chamomile	Dogwood
Flaxseed	Watermelon seed
Gum Arabic	Low mallows, apple, pear and quince gum, Balm, Watermelon seed
Ergot	Cotton-root
Guaiacum	Boxwood, Poke, Prickly ash
Ipecac	Wild Jalap, Carolina hipps

From civilwarhome.com/drugshsp

Medical Advances During the Civil War

The Civil War presented a great opportunity for physicians to learn about the various problems that occur as a consequence of battlefield injuries. Surgeons learned how to deal with simple and complicated injuries of the head, chest, abdomen, "ghastly wounds," and those of the vascular system. They learned how to ligate arteries better and more effectively in difficult lesions of the lower and upper extremities.

Surgeons were required to repair complicated injuries of the face. They began to use new plastic surgery techniques. To obtain the most appropriate closure of facial lesions, they had to be innovative and thereby developed the early secrets of good reconstructive surgery.

Surgeons were also forced to develop the most effective means of performing amputations. Amputations of all kinds, in various and difficult circumstances, were undertaken. Anesthesia was managed more consistently with excellent results and minimal morbidity and mortality. In spite of the advances in surgical procedure and technique reached during the Civil War, surgical knowledge was still significantly limited before the important developments of the 1880s.

The Civil War provided ample chance for developing an improved ambulance system. Medical transportation demanded the highest level of efficiency during this time period. The mobilization of the sick, the development of provisional hospitals (in particular the pavilion type), and improved embalming techniques were all advances seen during the Civil War. The Union also prospered in building hospitals, to such a degree that by the end of the war there were 204 Union general hospitals with beds for 136,894 patients. It was evident then, that this proved to be the maximum capacity for appropriate patient care.

Conclusion

The devastation from the Civil War was so extreme that at the time it might have appeared that more was lost than was won. More than half a million American compatriots died. Disease, mainly typhoid, dysentery, and pneumonia, killed more people than those who died in battle. When the war began, most of the surgeons and medical corps were unprepared, untrained, and uneducated. It was frequently said that the use of a laryngoscope, stethoscope, or ophthalmoscope by American physicians was a rarity. The use of hypodermic syringes to administer medicine had not reached clinical practice yet. All in all, a sad situation at this point in time.

At the end of this gruesome event, surgeons and medical personnel were better off because of it. Surgeons learned the best way to use anesthesia, to perform amputations, to ligate arteries, to operate on the vascular system, and to work on facial injuries. Mobilization of the sick and medical transportation was considerably improved. Hospital design improved. Embalming of the dead reached an art of highest degree.

During the years of the Civil War, medical science had not advanced to the point that antiseptic surgery was known, or the germ theory of the disease recognized, nor were sanitation and hygiene fully incorporated into routine clinical practice. Yet, physicians and medical practitioners did the best they could in the circumstances.

Great personalities such as those of Hammond and Letterman from the Union, Moore and Stout from the Confederacy, Bellows and Olmsted from the Sanitary Commission, and nurses Dix and Barton created an atmosphere of improvement and positive support for the rest of the medical corps and combatant soldiers. They brought new ideas, leadership skills, and a firm desire to do something about the appalling conditions they saw during the Civil War. There was no question that after the Civil War was over, they had reached their goals and much more!

CHAPTER 9
AMERICANS REJECT SCIENCE

John Duffy, noted American medical historian, summarized the skepticism of the late nineteenth century American physician: "Long after Pasteur and Koch had been acclaimed for their work, American physicians remained unconvinced." Indeed, Americans believed only in pragmatic solutions. In post-Civil War America, physicians still did not consider science as an important part of clinical medicine. They believed in practical ways or means to treat patients but not in theoretical explanations of the mechanisms of treating a particular disease. In this section, we review American physicians' lack of interest in science, particularly those living in the nineteenth century.

Utilitarian American Beliefs

American physicians recognized utilitarian means of life. However, if basic or clinical scientific research as exemplified by observation could not offer a clear and specific way of improving their medical or economic status, they were not interested in pursuing such an endeavor. Practicality and utility represented a unique way of viewing life. During the early years of the American nation, physicians needed to survive as members of an evolving profession, and they figured then that they could see the direct benefits of their treatments, therefore, science or the explanation of diseases would occupy a distant interest.

The American public was even more utilitarian in their way of viewing life than physicians were. In this ever-expanding young nation, there was not enough consideration for theory. Practical principles and ideas dominated the way of a society that began to take form. Survival was equal to practicality. Science was not considered high in the view and character of this skeptical nation.

The scientific successes encountered in Europe during the mid-nineteenth century did not impress utilitarian Americans. It was considered then that what was good for Europeans did not have a direct application to the American way of doing things, unless these concepts had a practical use. Americans also understood that in order to survive, they needed more than science. Up to the 1880s, Americans did not make a full association between medical science and technology; otherwise, they would have completely accepted science since they were firm believers in the practical applications of technology.

As the last third of the nineteenth century progressed close to the 1890s, the American public and American physicians began to reconsider their utilitarian position. They started to draw attention to the fact that science and research were not against a utilitarian point of view. In fact, it seemed obvious to them that both concepts, science and utilitarianism, would be greatly expanded if both areas could be utilized to improve each other. The American medical mind was making efforts at accepting plausible scientific principles as well as interwoven science, technology, and practice.

Simplicity Negates Science

Benjamin Rush (1745-1813) (Figure 4), the American Hippocrates, considered the father of American medicine, and a dominant force in the field for many years, was responsible for creating an ambience of simplicity in the practice of medicine. He proposed a single cause for all diseases; he enunciated once, "Where I formerly said there was only one fever, I will now say there is but one disease in the world." Rush concluded that the source of all illness was vascular tension. Therefore, for him, the way to relieve tension was to produce bleeding. He was certainly true to his principles since his avocation and support of bleeding for all diseases constantly permeated his whole life.

During the first third of the nineteenth century, medical ideas and practice were under Rush's influence. The heroic medicine of bleeding, purging, and emetics for all diseases was the rule. One treatment for all diseases equaled simplicity, lack of inquisitiveness, and little interest in research and science. Though Rush was considered a hero in American medicine, he also played an important role in the retardation of the acceptance of scientific principles in this country.

Years after Rush's death, physicians continued to apply his concepts of "desperate remedies for desperate diseases" (Duffy). Wisely, the public began to oppose the dismal effects of this ill-conceived therapy. The simplistic approach to medicine – one cause for everything and one treatment for all – was not working!

In the 1870s, there were some physicians who were still recommending heroic measures. By the 1880s, more physicians recognized the importance of science in the practice of medicine, and the simplistic approach to disease began to disappear. By the 1890s, the idea of one cause for all diseases and one treatment had faded. Science began a rapid ascending path which has continued even until our days.

Opposition to the Germ Theory of the Disease

In 1877, Rudolf Virchow (1821-1902), distinguished German pathologist, indicated his point of view as far as science and medicine was concerned:

> It is no longer necessary today to write that scientific medicine is also the best foundation for medical practice. It is sufficient to point out how completely even the external character of medical practice has changed in the last thirty years. Scientific methods have been everywhere introduced into practice. The diagnosis and prognosis of the physician are based on the experience of the pathological anatomist and the physiologist. Therapeutic doctrine has become biological and thereby experimental science.

The same was not true in the United States. In the same year, American physicians and surgeons rejected Lister's antiseptic method, which was based on the germ theory of the disease. Only a few American surgeons accepted this method. Among them, Robert Weir, a recognized New York surgeon pointed out the lack of interest of American surgeons in the Listerian principles of wound management. In 1878, Moritz Schuppert, a New Orleans surgeon, published 120 operations with considerably improved results using Lister's methods. Immediately after these findings, Schuppert retired and the method was no longer practiced at the New Orleans Charity Hospital. In 1887, Frederick Parham reintroduced it, when a bout of puerperal fever was discovered in the surgical wards.

Other American surgeons did not receive Listerian principles with enthusiasm. The failure to recognize germs as the cause of surgical infections was a failure to appreciate the scientific basis of disease and a lack of acceptance for the science behind medicine. At this stage of their evolution, American physicians did not consider science an important part of medical practice. In the 1890s, everything changed. Everything became enlightened with scientific principles; everything represented a well-defined cause-and-effect relationship in the realization of medical treatments; everything was conceived to accept the science introduced by our European counterparts. Finally, a new age where science explained disease began to spread through the United States!

Opposition to Research

Bordley and Harvey, in narrating the odyssey of *Two Centuries of American Medicine* in 1976, summarized their perceptions of the first century of medicine (1776-1876) of this new nation:

> There was no systematic research and very little research of any type during the first century. The American contributions to medical progress...were concerned for the most part with the natural history of diseases or with improvements in surgical methods. In only a few instances were experiments involved.

The experimental interest of American physicians was not evident during a great part of the nineteenth century. Few exceptions of notable Americans had demonstrated their concern for scientific discovery. An extraordinary exception of a gifted individual who believed in the inventive potential of the American mind was Benjamin Franklin (1706-1790). Louis Pasteur (1822-1895), the famous French scientist, is quoted as saying:

> Without theory, practice is but the routine born of habit. Theory alone can bring forth and develop the spirit of invention. It is to you specially that it will belong not to share the opinion of those narrow minds who disdain everything in science which has no immediate application. You know Franklin's charming saying? He was witnessing the first demonstration of a purely scientific discovery, and the people round him said: 'But what is the use of it?' Franklin answered them: 'What is the use of a new-born child?' (Bordley and Harvey)

Other significant exceptions to the lack of interest in research by American physicians during the first half of the nineteenth century were William Beaumont (1785-1853), who in the 1820s performed classical experiments outlining gastric secretion, and Samuel D. Gross (1805-1884), who in 1840 conducted experimental studies on wounds of the intestines in dogs. The rest of American physicians working in medical schools or in private practice were not that interested or found it difficult to establish clinical or animal research studies in the United States.

Physicians of the 1870s and 1880s still had little interest in research. This appeared to be different for non-medical American scientists. Noted American science historian Robert Bruce indicates in his Pulitzer Prize winning book, *The Launching of Modern American Science, 1846-1876*, that American scientists saw the mid-nineteenth century (1846-1876) as the period when the "ideas, needs, and directions of these scientists began to coalesce, and the organized, truly national, and highly professional community that we know today was established." The development of medical science and research was different since physicians did not appear to show consistent interest in research or science until the 1890s. Few and isolated events had appeared before this decade but nothing that amounted to a systematic approach to medical research sciences. It is possible to assume, then, that non-medical American scientists had a different way of seeing their particular disciplines as compared to the American physicians of the time. Physicians were reluctant to accept research and, therefore, to accept science in the practice of medicine.

Lack of Education and Academic Standards

The status of American medical education during a great part of the nineteenth century was disastrous. Few principles and theories of disease were being taught, and no real academic standards were in practice. American physicians cared little about education and academic goals. They attended medical school to complete the minimal requirements to practice medicine. They were not interested in finding explanations for the causes of diseases nor reasons for the types of treatments. They were not committed to academic pursuits or the development of research-related studies. They were focused in practical endeavors conducive to practical and simple results.

In the mid-nineteenth century, the popular image of the medical profession was low. According to Duffy,

> Those who could afford to go to college and medical school, and then on to Europe to complete their medical training, were usually the ones who held the best positions as medical professors and enjoyed the most lucrative practices...Below this top group were a fairly large number of physicians holding reputable medical degrees who were able to make a comfortable living...Still further down the social and economic scale was the large number of

> physicians whose training was derived from an apprenticeship or from one of the many second- and third-rate medical schools...Many of them were barely literate, a situation which did little to enhance the reputation of the profession.

In a review of physicians practicing in 1847, Miller recognized the discouraging status of the medical profession. In the state of Virginia, almost 25% of the practicing physicians had neither medical degree nor license. "In the new states west of the Appalachians where life was even more freewheeling, it was estimated that half of the practitioners had no formal qualifications." Other distinguished physician writers of the time such as Daniel Drake (1785-1852) reported similar or worse conditions associated with the practice of medicine in mid-nineteenth century America. As if this were not enough, Duffy continues by mentioning three important reasons for the difficulties faced by American physicians of the mid-nineteenth century: (1) the lack of medical knowledge in general, (2) constant quarrelling among physicians, and (3) the need for some basic principles that would explain the causes of diseases.

In the second half of the nineteenth century, the medical scene had scarcely changed. In the 1870s, President Eliot at Harvard and Nathan Davis in Chicago were asking for reforms in medical education. It was clear then that medical students did not have the discipline and character found in the students of other schools. Only a few medical schools such as Harvard, Northwestern, Syracuse, Pennsylvania, and Michigan were joining the efforts of adopting a graded three-year curriculum, even though the educational requirements for admission were virtually nonexistent. Between 1867 and 1876, 21 new orthodox medical schools and 5 homeopathic schools were founded, most of them with "the poorest quality, thus serving to depress the average level of competence of medical school graduates" (Bordley and Harvey).

As late as 1876, the well-known British scientist, Thomas Huxley, spoke in Baltimore about the poor quality of students admitted into medical schools, that they did not have a concept of the physical sciences, and that for the first time they realized that sciences such as physics, chemistry, and physiology existed. "Much of the first session is wasted in learning how to learn,...and in awakening their dormant and wholly untrained powers of observation and manipulation" (Bordley and Harvey). Huxley continued to emphasize the lack of scientific training in the existing system of education. William Welch, distinguished pathologist, medical educator, and future dean of Johns Hopkins Medical School, concurred with Huxley's observations and stated that as he graduated from college at Yale (1870) and medical school at Columbia (1875), he noted "the inadequate preliminary requirements, the short courses, the faulty arrangement of the curriculum, the dominance of the didactic lecture, the meager appliances for demonstrative and practical instruction" (Bordley and Harvey).

As far as 1889, William Osler, at the time professor of Medicine at the University of Pennsylvania, eloquently spoke about the shameful state of affairs of the American Medical System in general:

> It makes one's blood boil to think that there are sent out year by year scores of men called doctors, who have never attended a case of labor, and who are utterly ignorant of the ordinary everyday diseases which they may be called upon to treat; men who may never have seen the inside of a hospital ward and who would not know Scarpa's space from the sole of the foot. Yet, gentlemen, this is the disgraceful condition which some school-men have the audacity to ask you to perpetuate; to continue to entrust interests so sacred to hands so unworthy. Is it to be wondered, considering this shocking laxity, that there is a widespread distrust in the public of professional education, and that quacks, charlatans and imposters possess the land? (Bordley and Harvey)

By the 1890s, medical education began to improve in a few leading schools in the United States: Harvard, Pennsylvania, Michigan, and Minnesota. Hopkins was in the process of hiring its faculty with Welch being the first professor named in 1884. The school did not open until 1893. The Association of American Medical Colleges, which had been founded in 1876, had been inactive for a few years before it was reinvigorated when Hopkins began its effort to change medical education. In 1910, Abraham Flexner published his monumental report on *Medical Education in the United States and Canada*. Based on his survey of all schools, this report is considered the decisive document that changed medical education and the course of medicine forever.

Conclusion

American physicians rejected science during most of the nineteenth century. The reasons behind this position could be explained by: 1) utilitarian beliefs, 2) simplicity, 3) opposition to the germ theory of the disease, 4) opposition to research, and 5) lack of education and academic standards. The 1890s marked the most important decade into the final acceptance of science and research-related matters by the American physician in particular and the public in general.

CHAPTER 10
KNIFE AT WORK AND THE BUGS WHAT

Before the nineteenth century, anesthesia did not exist in the United States of America or the rest of the world. Surgery was, in essence, primitive and no elaborate procedures could be performed because of the untreated effect of pain. Surgeons had to proceed swiftly with their operations, which basically amounted to cutting extremities, draining abscesses, ligating bleeding vessels, and removing superficial tumors. It was a very limited field of practice, something that was about to change in the near future

This section analyzes the state of surgery in the United States, particularly around the nineteenth century, and investigates the important role that the germ theory of disease played in surgical practice.

Early American Surgeons

Zabdiel Boylston (1679-1766) performed the first elective surgical operation in English America during colonial times (1607-1783). Boylston had been born and educated in Massachusetts. He had attended an apprenticeship with John Cutter of Boston and did not attend medical school in Europe or on the American continent since one had not been founded there yet. On June 24, 1710, he extracted a bladder stone in a child. The notice of such an operation appeared in the Boston News-Letter of July 17-24, 1710, and apparently was the third one he had performed for this ailment. Another operation, a breast amputation for cancer, one of the earliest operations for cancer in the colonies, appeared in the Boston Gazette of November 21-28, 1720, not an easy undertaking for surgery without anesthesia!

Sylvester Gardiner (1707-1786) from Rhode Island, John Bard (1716-1799) from New Jersey, John Jones (1729-1791) from New York, James

Robertson (1742-1814) from Virginia, and John Hartshorn (1735-?) and James Thatcher (1754-1844) from Massachusetts all made important contributions to surgery prior to the nineteenth century. Table 10.1 denotes the type of contributions they made.

Table 10.1. Pioneering Contributions of Early American Surgeons to the Development of Surgery

Surgeon	Year	Contribution
Zabdiel Boylston	1710	Removal of Bladder Stone Amputation of Breast for Cancer
Sylvester Gardiner	1741	Removal of Bladder Stone
John Hartshorn	1752	Detailed Description of Leg Dressings, Sinus Formation, Abscess Drainage, and Amputation
John Bard	1760	Extraction of Infected Uterine Fetus
John Jones	1775	First American Textbook on Military and Trauma Surgery
James Thatcher	1775	Began Military Surgical Diary (until 1783)
James Robertson	1777	Management of Scalped Head

Nineteenth Century American Surgeons Prior to 1846

From the end of colonial times until the discovery of anesthesia in the United States in 1846, the practice of surgery continued to be clearly limited. There were no elective procedures being performed and surgeons and patients shied away from them, too much suffering to be tolerated by prospective patients. Few of them were willing to proceed with surgery. Avoidance was the rule.

Few surgeons attempted to perform complicated surgical procedures. Morbidity and mortality were frequent companions of those surgeries undertaken in spite of the lack of anesthesia. Not having enough time limited the opportunity for maximizing the surgeon's ability to perform a good operation. Time represented better results. Anesthesia, therefore, represented better surgery and the performance of cases with complicated situations. Distinguished surgeons, even before the advent of anesthesia, decided to operate on some difficult cases. Table 10.2 reflects the surgeon, the time, and the pioneering role that he played in some of the advances of surgery of the times.

Rothstein, noted medical historian, addressed the importance of anesthesia in the practice of surgery during the first half of the nineteenth century:

The lack of anesthesia was the most terrifying surgical problem before the second half of the nineteenth century. Patients refused or delayed surgery if at all possible; tumors, for example, were allowed to grow to fifty or one hundred pounds before removal. Surgical operations themselves reflected the horror of the event.

Table 10.2. Pioneering Contributions of American Surgeons from the End of the Colonial Period (1783) to the Discovery of Anesthesia (1846)

Surgeon	Year	Contribution
Thomas Smith*	1805	Experimental intestinal suture
Samuel White	1806	Removal of spoon from intestine
Ephraim McDowell (Figure 10)	1809	Extirpation of enlarged ovarian cyst
John Syng Dorsey	1811	Tie off femoral artery for aneurysms Removal of bladder stone
Philip Syng Physick[†]	1812 1816	Extracting poisonous substance from stomach Use of animal sutures
Valentine Mott	1818	Ligature of inominate artery
Nathan Smith	1821 1822	Extraction of foreign substances from esophagus Removal of ovary for dropsy
William Beaumont (Figure 11)	1822	Gastric secretion studies
Benjamin Dudley	1823[‡]	Management of head injuries, trephining the cranium
Aquila Toland	1837	Suture of intestine and omentum
Henry Beach	•	Case reports of Massachusetts General Hospital before 1846
John Collins Warren	1846	First demonstration of effective use of ether in surgery

*Not American citizen, from St. Croix Islands, studying at University of Pennsylvania.
†Multiple other contributions by Physick are not included here.
‡Date of publication.
•Paper published in 1897.

John Collins Warren (1778-1856), the outstanding Boston surgeon who performed the first major surgical operation under ether, would see the operative procedure in the following way:

> In case of amputation, it was the custom to bring the patient into the operating room and place him upon the table. [The surgeon] would stand with his hands behind his back and would say to the patient, 'Will you have your leg off or will you not have it off?' If the patient lost courage and said, 'No,' he had decided not to have the leg amputated, he was at once carried back to his bed in the

> ward. If, however, he said, 'Yes,' he was immediately taken firmly in hand by a number of strong assistants and the operation went on regardless of whatever he might say thereafter. If his courage failed him after this crucial moment, it was too late and no attention was paid to his cries of protest. It was found to be the only practicable method by which an operation could be performed under the gruesome conditions which prevailed before the advent of anesthesia.

American Surgeons from 1846 to 1867

After the introduction of anesthesia in 1846 and the publication of Lister's pioneering work in 1867, American surgeons and those around the world began to have more flexibility in approaching surgical procedures and solving cases that were unreachable before. Even though anesthesia had given better opportunities of success for surgeons and patients alike, a formidable enemy had not been conquered. Infection, the presence of germs, had not been dominated and was the source of significant morbidity and mortality of surgical patients. The use of antiseptics had existed much before the nineteenth century and "surgeons applied these techniques in all contaminated wounds." In another work, we previously summarized the conditions of wound management before Joseph Lister's (1827-1912) seminal contribution of 1867:

> There was no clear understanding of the principles of wound management and the reasons their methods succeeded. The atmosphere was ready for new achievements in the basic sciences to permit a complete understanding of all these empirical applications. (Toledo-Pereyra, *Amer J Surg*)

Even before the germs were appropriately controlled by strict Listerian techniques, James Marion Sims (1813-1883) performed his first successful operation for vesico-vaginal fistula in Montgomery, Alabama, in 1849. This case was followed by a series of cases with equal degrees of success. Sims was not the first to correct this defect, but he was the one who "devised a successful and reproducible operation." Other surgeons continued to perform different operations even though poor resources and results limited the outcomes because of infected surgical wounds.

During the Civil War (1861-1865), surgeons enhanced their experience by operating on a large number of soldiers with battlefield injuries. Amputations of various sizes and locations, wound injuries, and multiple vascular damage were frequently seen in the population at risk. Antiseptics were being used in various forms and types, but nothing that similated the antiseptic system of Lister. At the end of this cruel event, mortality had reached incredible proportions, in part due to battlefield injuries and in part due to surgical infections. Better means of wound management, according to Lister's method, were not available just yet. In Glasgow, Scotland, Lister did his first case under his antiseptic techniques on August 12, 1865, and published his first eleven cases in *Lancet* in 1867. American surgeons had not had enough time, up to this point, to recognize and readily accept Lister's principles. They were skeptical in accepting a system that appeared to be complicated and, according to them, not offering a significant advantage over their own system. Time and the belief in the germ theory would change their way of thinking!

Semmelweis – Pasteur – Koch – Lister

Completely separate from the United States, before 1865, Europe had made significant contributions in the field of antisepsis and the germ theory of the disease. Ignaz Semmelweis (1818-1865) in 1847, in Vienna, introduced the chlorine hand washing technique and sanitation of clothes and instruments to diminish the incidence of puerperal fever after delivery of pregnant patients. In 1857, Louis Pasteur (1822-1895), a French *bona fide* chemist, who solved important chemical and biological problems, began to solidify the germ theory, when demonstrated, through a series of well-planned experiments, that germs were responsible for fermentation.

In 1860, Lemaire, a French medical scientist, introduced carbolic acid in medicine and surgery. In 1865, Lister began a series of cases, of compound fractures and wound infections, where the use of carbolic acid significantly decreased mortality and, therefore, confirmed the role of germs in the development of surgical diseases such as pyemia, erysipelas, and hospital gangrene. It was apparent at this time in history that the successful application of previous discoveries culminated in the comprehensive utilization by Lister of this scientific knowledge. He was able to translate science into clinical practice in a way that others could not do. Because of this, he should be considered the father of antiseptic surgery, particularly because he was able to apply his method, under the new principles, of what would be the germ theory of disease.

Robert Koch (1843-1910), German bacteriologist, around 1876 culminated a series of studies that demonstrated the important role of germs in the development of disease. He introduced four postulates that confirmed the presence of germs as the cause of disease. Finally, at this point, belief in the germ theory of the disease had been fully and completely integrated into the medical scene!

Lister's Method in More Detail

Lister was extremely meticulous and rigorous in the application of his antiseptic surgical technique. He followed very closely and with tedious detail the most intricate parts of the procedure. In a previous paper, referring to *A Critical Study of Lister's Work on Antiseptic Surgery*, we presented a brief description of Lister's method. In Lister's own words, he said:

> I first washed the skin of the forearm and elbow with 1 to 20 watery solution of carbolic acid, to destroy all putrefactive particles in the epidermis and hair follicles, and then made a longitudinal incision about two inches long over the back of the ulna where it had been broken, while an assistant threw over the part a cloud of spray of 1 to 40 carbolic lotion by means of Richardson's apparatus...I inserted the blades of a pair of strong bone-pliers, smeared with an oil solution of acid (1 to 10)...A sponge wrung out of 1 to 40 water solution having then been bandaged upon the wound...

Lister achieved superb results with his method. Mortality decreased from 45 to 15 percent. Cheyne, a disciple of Lister, reported even better results, when he indicated that only 5% of patients treated antiseptically died. Lister's antiseptic system was strictly based on the germ theory of disease, even at a time when this important concept had not been fully accepted. There were several principles on which the whole method of Lister had been supported: 1) germs needed to be eliminated before or after surgery, 2) germs surrounding the wound needed to be destroyed, 3) germs in the wound should not be spread, and 4) instruments, dressings, and surgeon's hands should be washed with carbolic acid.

Lister continued to study the effect of germs suspended in the atmosphere. In 1871, he published a work reviewing how putrefactive changes in the vehicle utilized (wine in this case) were caused by particles of dust suspended in the atmosphere. Lister pursued this work to unravel the origins of wound infections. His work was indispensable in confirming the role of microorganisms in the infectious process. He investigated, in a detailed moment, the overall effect of germs in wound infections. He was a significant source of information for those believing in the germ theory of disease.

American Surgeons After 1867 and the Practice of Listerism

In 1867, when Lister's work was widely recognized by the medical and scientific world because of his *Lancet* publication, American surgeons were not prepared to subscribe to his theories. American practitioners of surgery believed in Lister's results but were not committing themselves to the acceptance of the germ theory of disease. They felt that the principles of Listerism were too complicated to be utilized in practical surgery. There appeared to have been a misunderstanding between the proclaimed system and the understood explanation of it. Almost two decades will have to occur prior to complete acceptance of Listerism.

In 1876, nine years after the publication of Lister's main paper and at the time of the 5th International Medical Congress in Philadelphia, Lister had the opportunity to explain Listerism to his American audience. Some took detailed notes and began to show some interest; others such as Samuel D. Gross (1805-1884) (Figure 12) from Philadelphia were not convinced of such a system. Candid discussions arose from the meeting, and no clear winner emerged from this event. The English surgeon did his best in explaining his system, and the American surgical group showed no evidence of considering the Listerian principles in high esteem.

The great American professor, Samuel Gross, was not ready to accept Listerian practices. We have previously summarized Gross' beliefs in Listerism:

> Gross outlined his opposition to antiseptic principles. He knew all about Pasteur's research on the presence of minute organisms in the atmosphere that had been invoked as a cause of wound contamination. Gross, however, was very reluctant to believe in the germ theory of disease (Toledo-Pereyra, 1976). Although he used antiseptics for open abscesses, wounds, and compound fractures, he was not convinced of their usefulness. He thought that the use of antiseptics did not change the outcome of the open abscess. Gross used antiseptics merely to arrest the process of putrefaction and to destroy its products. According to Pasteur's concept, the atmosphere was filled with invisible living germs which, coming into contact with the putrescible material of open wounds, induced putrefaction and irritation. The aim of Lister's antiseptic treatment, therefore, was to destroy the septic potential of germs in the atmosphere. For Gross the interpretation of this phenomenon was different: 'the atmosphere of ill-ventilated and

> long-occupied hospitals contains a noxious, invisible, permeable dust, holding in suspension epithelial and pus cells which is capable by direct contact with wounded surface to induce putrefaction and blood-poisoning through its absorption by the lungs' (Sigerist). From a practical point of view Gross' opinion altered the surgeon's private practice. Gross' experience in private practice caused him to treat primary wounds by simple closure, to open abscesses, and to unite compound fractures, but he did not take special antiseptic care or any other measure to prevent would contamination. (Toledo-Peryera, *Current Surgery*)

In 1877, Robert F. Weir, a New York city surgeon, outlined the reasons for American surgeons' slow acceptance of Listerism. The continuous changes by Lister, the need for supervision by the practicing surgeon, and the enunciation of the germ theory of disease as the basis for Lister's theories were all causes for tardiness in the acceptance of Listerism. Around the same time, Robert Koch published an important work on the etiology of traumatic infective diseases that opened up a significant opportunity for the acceptance of Lister's principles.

By 1882, barely five years later, Professor Gross was going to write on the 6th edition of his *System of Surgery* that he had changed his mind on Listerism. He now accepted its practice even though he still was not near to believing in the germ theory. During the same year, at the American Surgical Association meeting, W. T. Briggs from Nashville discussed the antiseptic treatment of wounds but did not fully accept the germ theory. Other surgeons such as B. A. Watson from New Jersey had the same beliefs. Contrarily, C. B. Nancrede, initially from Philadelphia and later from Michigan, completely believed in Listerism and the germ theory of disease. By the mid-1880s, there was complete acceptance of the germ theory of disease in the United States of America. By now, Listerism was beyond non-belief and surgeons would not challenge its value any longer! Surgeons were part of a large group of believers.

Other notable American surgeons during this time included: Henry Jacob Bigelow (1816-1890) from Harvard in Boston, the first American to resect the hip joint; D. Hayes Agnew (1818-1892) (Figure 13) from the University of Pennsylvania in Philadelphia, who performed many pioneering surgical techniques; Nicholas Senn (1844-1909), from Rush Medical College in Chicago who undertook significant abdominal surgery work; Stephen Smith from New York, who maintained the great importance of cleanliness in all operations; and the group of Reginald H. Fitz (1843-1913) from Boston, Charles McBurney (1845-1913) from New York, and L. L. McArthur from Chicago who all had done pioneering work on the diagnosis and pathogenesis of appendicitis. William W. Keen (1837-1932) from Philadelphia; Rudolph Matas from New Orleans; George Crile (1864-1943) from Cleveland; William S. Halsted (1852-1922) from Baltimore; and John B Murphy (1857-1916) from Chicago also made significant surgical contributions in the latter part of the nineteenth century and beginning of the twentieth century. American surgery was indeed on its way to a site of notoriety and excellence in the world.

Conclusion

American surgery of the nineteenth century could be divided into three phases: before 1846—the time of the discovery of ether anesthesia for major surgical operations; between 1846 and 1867—the time of the publication of Lister's work based on antiseptic principles according to Lister; and after 1867—the time of the acceptance of Listerism and the germ theory of disease. Americans did not readily accept Lister's concepts because of their changing nature, the requirement for supervision, and the importance of believing in the germ theory. American surgeons, then, did not believe in the germ theory of disease until the latter part of the nineteenth century. By the mid-1880s, practically all American surgeons had embraced the significance of germs in the cause of infections associated with surgical operations. From here on, antisepsis for the American surgeon was based on the germ theory of disease.

CHAPTER 11
HOPKINS TAKES THE LEAD

In 1893, the first modern medical school in the United States was founded. Johns Hopkins Medical School represented a modern institution following the ideas and principles of the best European institutions. They modeled themselves after German medical schools with full-time faculty, bedside teaching, participation in laboratory instruction, and the possibility of research, a unique opportunity for young American students. This section analyzes the development of Johns Hopkins Medical School as a modern medical school established at the end of the nineteenth century and reviews the circumstances surrounding this major event.

Preambles to Johns Hopkins Medical School

After the US Civil War, three medical schools, Harvard, Pennsylvania, and Michigan, began to structure themselves in a way that was going to modernize them and make them more competitive in the American medical education arena. President Charles W. Eliot from Harvard, provosts Charles Stillé and William Pepper, Jr., from Pennsylvania, and president James B. Angell from Michigan were all decisive elements on creating change and improving medical education in their own universities and medical schools.

At Harvard, Eliot began by exerting more control over the medical school. In 1869, after taking over the presidency of the university, he assumed full responsibilities for the medical faculty as well as, on his own desire, became the chair of the faculty, a position he maintained for the next forty years. In 1871, wit the help of his allies, Eliot succeeded in realizing a series of reforms in the medical school. The antagonistic views of his dissenters, Oliver Wendell Holmes and Henry Jacob Bigelow, did not prevail. The changes included: 1) the medical school became an integral part of the university with fees and salaries handled by the university; 2) the course of instruction was expanded to a three-year program with nine-month terms and written exams for all subjects; and 3) emphasis on laboratory sciences. Henry Pickering Bowditch became the first professor of physiology in the United States to devote himself full-time to teaching and research. Other reforms came about in subsequent years (Table 11.1).

Eliot's plan of emphasizing the scientific principles by the students' "learning by doing" was perhaps the most notable development of the reforms of 1871. Eliot believed, following German influence, that

> science (should be) taught in a rational way, objects and instruments at hand – not from books merely, not through memory chiefly, but by the seeing eye and the informing fingers.

On the heels of Harvard, the University of Pennsylvania began pushing for reform. In 1877, the medical school changed its course structure and overall curriculum, extending it to three years, making tuition paid directly to the university and requiring examination for the attended subjects. S. Weir Mitchell, strong supporter of the reforms, had become a member of the board of trustees of the university in 1876. Immediately thereafter, he was named chairman of the board's medical committee, a position he kept for the next 35 years. The changes at Pennsylvania were very similar to what had happened at Harvard (Table 11.1).

The University of Michigan did not wait long either. With the support of President Angell and the tireless commitment of Dean Victor Vaughn, Michigan concentrated on the teaching of sciences throughout the curriculum. Vaughn, a biochemist, had spent some time in Germany with the famed Robert Koch, where he learned the importance of science and research in the development of modern and more efficient medical schools. He began the Michigan reforms in 1877 by increasing the annual sessions from six to nine months and in 1880 by expanding the curriculum to three years. Ten years later, a fourth year became obligatory (Table 11.1). Vaughn appointed key faculty to Michigan, a group of eminent medical scientists who had had German academic exposure: physiologists Henry Sewall, William Howell, and Warren Lombard; anatomist Frank Mall; pharmacologists John J. Abel and Arthur Cushny; chemist Paul Freer; and bacteriologist Frederick Novi. This faculty was prepared to make Michigan's medical school respected.

Table 11.1. Important Dates in Medical Education of the Leading US Medical Schools of the Late Nineteenth Century

	Harvard	Pennsylvania	Michigan	Hopkins
1871	3-year curriculum			
1877		3-year curriculum, practical instruction of sciences	6-month term changed to 9-month	
1880	Optional 4th year		3-year curriculum, All students lab instructed	
1882		5-month term changed to 6-month		
1883		Optional 4th year		
1890			Mandatory 4th year	
1892	Mandatory 4th year			
1893		Mandatory 4th year		Founded first modern medical school, Bachelor of Science degree required, 4-year curriculum, Full-time faculty
1900	Bachelor degree required			

Kenneth Ludmerer, well-known medical education historian, referred to the Michigan Medical School in the following way:

> By the early 1890s, Michigan had become, in the opinion of many, the strongest scientific medical school in the country. Vaughn proudly reminded readers in his autobiography that of the original eight full professors of the Johns Hopkins Medical School in 1893, four had Michigan degrees and two were taken directly from the Michigan faculty.

The reforms put in motion at Harvard, Pennsylvania and Michigan were the preliminary steps for the beginning of the best medical school education in the world. To this, the most incredible experiment in medical education would occur in Baltimore, the unique creation of the Johns Hopkins Medical School in 1893, which we will describe next.

Founding of Johns Hopkins University

The generosity, vision, and extraordinary desire of Johns Hopkins to create something particularly unique strongly motivated him to found the greatest medical experiment on record. His fortune of seven million dollars was donated in 1867 to build a university, a hospital, and a medical school that eventually would be responsible for the hospital operations.

Johns Hopkins was a bachelor who had amassed his fortune from the railroad business and who had limitless generosity. How he came up with this idea is not completely clear since his interest in education and medical sciences was not well-known. There was no doubt, however, in his specific commitment to this cause. It is here, perhaps, where we can let Bordley and Harvey's exceptional book entitled *Two Centuries of American Medicine* present to us their assessment of Mr. Hopkins' circumstances involved in his extraordinary donation:

> No one knows just how Johns Hopkins acquired the knowledge that enabled him to plan so wisely for the role which his university and hospital were to play in reforming medical education in the United States. He was a man of limited education, none of it professional, and he had devoted his life to the world of business. Nevertheless, when he devised his bequest in 1867 for a university medical school and a hospital with interlocking boards of Trustees, he recognized the importance, which was then only dimly perceived by many medical educators, of having a medical school organized as an integral department of a university and of having the clinical education of medical students carried out in a hospital closely connected with the medical school. It is believed, on the basis of circumstantial evidence, that Patrick Macauley, a physician who lived near Mr. Hopkins in Baltimore, may have influenced the latter's views. In 1823, Macauley addressed the Medical and Chirurgical Faculty of Maryland on the subject of Medical Improvement. In this address he dwelt upon the use of hospitals for clinical instruction. Macauley died in 1849. From 1847 to 1849 he and Hopkins served together on the Board of Directors of the Baltimore and Ohio Railroad. Whether Macauley ever discussed medical education with Hopkins is not known; but it is of interest that Mr. Hopkins's library was found, after his death, to contain books on medical subjects which had belonged to

Dr. Macauley.

After Johns Hopkins' death in 1873 and following the specific wishes expressed in his will, the executors began to bring about each and every one of his recommended actions. The first order of business was for securing a president for the new university. In 1876, Daniel C. Gilman was imported from the University of California at Berkeley, where he was their current president. As soon as he arrived, he began the recruitment of individuals who would participate in the hospital design and construction as well as those who subsequently began the planning of the medical school.

Gilman, in his new position, was responsible for the university's growth. He selected exceptional individuals to head the science departments: H. Newell Martin in Biology, Henry A. Rowland in Physics, and Ira Remsen in Chemistry. These men represented the best that science could offer in the United States, all young, well-prepared, and with an enormous desire to teach and accomplish the best. With their advice and that of John Shaw Billings (1839-1913) in medical matters, the university and later on the hospital and medical school were in apt and dedicated hands.

Development of Johns Hopkins Hospital

Johns Hopkins in his 1867 will requested that the new hospital should have its own board of trustees independent from the university board of trustees. His intention was to secure a position for the hospital within the university. In a letter in 1873, he addressed the trustees of the hospital in the following manner:

> It will be your special duty to secure for the service of the hospital surgeons and physicians of the highest character and of the greatest skill. I desire you to establish in connection with the hospital a training school for female nurses.
>
> In all your arrangements in relation to this hospital you will bear constantly in mind that it is my wish and purpose that the institution should ultimately form a part of the medical school of that university for which I have made ample provision in my will.

In 1875, before President Gilman had taken office, the hospital trustees sent a letter to hospital construction experts to determine the best plan for the development of the Johns Hopkins Hospital. Among the plans submitted, the one by John Shaw Billings was clearly the best. Billings had had a long military history as an organizer, administrator, and competent surgeon. His study on *Army Barracks and Hospitals* published in 1870 and his previous experience in the Civil War and thereafter made him one of the country's leading authorities on hospital design and construction. He had received his MD from the Medical College of Ohio in 1860 and taught anatomy and entered practice in Cincinnati. In 1861, he joined the army for a long and committed career.

From 1876 to 1889, Billings coordinated all details associated with the construction of the Johns Hopkins Hospital (Figure 14). During this time, Billings continued as officer of the army in charge of the Surgeon General's Library (now the National Library of Medicine). On May 7, 1889, the hospital was formally opened with President Gilman as its first director since Billings had refused the position of administrative director. Later the same year, Henry M. Hurd assumed this important position at Hopkins. He had received his BA and MD from the University of Michigan and had worked in the Michigan Asylum at Kalamazoo and the Eastern Michigan Asylum at Pontiac where in 1878 he became its first superintendent. In this last occupation, he demonstrated excellent administrative ability. President Angell from Michigan had already written Gilman a letter of recommendation where he emphasized about Hurd:

> I think it would be no mistake if you should appoint him...We have tried more than once to persuade him to take a medical chair here. He is refined, scholarly, gentlemanly, conciliatory in manner, capable of managing men pleasantly. He is a man of noble and elevated character.

Hurd's long-term commitment to Hopkins had even better results than what President Angell had indicated in his letter of support. Hopkins attracted personalities like Hurd who gave a great deal of recognition and strength to the institution (Table 11.2).

Integration of Johns Hopkins Medical School

In 1885, William H. Welch began his work as professor of Pathology at Johns Hopkins University. He was the first faculty hired for the new medical school, which had not yet been built or organized. With high hopes and abundant dreams, Welch began to appoint the clinical faculty. He included William Osler from the University of Pennsylvania, William S. Halsted from the College of Physicians and Surgeons at New York, and Howard A. Kelly from the University of Pennsylvania. All were affectionately known, after the extraordinary painting by John Singer Sargent (1856-1925), as *The Four Doctors* (Figure 15).

Table 11.2. Significant Events in the Development of Johns Hopkins University and Medical School	
Date	Event
1867	Johns Hopkins'' will designates $7 million* to be divided equally between a hospital and a medical school
1875	Daniel C. Gilman named as first president
1876	Johns Hopkins University begins
1876-1889	John Shaw Billings designs and supervises hospital construction
1885	William H. Welch begins as professor of pathology
1886-1889	Halsted works in Welch's labs
1889	Johns Hopkins Hospital opens
1893	Medical School opens
*Approximately $50 billion today, if one considers that the initial bequest of $7 million doubled every ten years between 1867 and 2004. In any event, a large sum of money under any economic estimation.	

Once the clinical sciences were secured, Gilman, Billings, and Welch (serving as dean of the medical school) had the responsibility of attracting young and promising candidates to head the basic sciences. Franklin P. Mall in anatomy, John Jacob Abel in pharmacology and physiological chemistry, and William H. Howell in physiology had all received an MD or PhD from the University of Michigan. Dr. Hurd, the hospital administrator had also received an MD from the same university. This reflected a strong connection between the medical schools of Michigan and Hopkins (Table 11.3), a collaboration that would continue in the years to come!

Close to the opening of the medical school, a group of women, headed by Mary E. Garrett, secured a total endowment of nearly $500,000 for the medical school with the provision that women would be considered for acceptance on the same terms as men. The board of trustees accepted the final offer, and when the medical school opened in 1893, women were admitted with the first and subsequent classes.

Finally, the medical school was in full force. In the fall of 1893, the first class consisted of 17 students, including three women. All of them were college graduates with an emphasis on the basic sciences and modern languages. It was an ideal group that was going to receive a four-year graded curriculum, two years of pre-clinical studies and, thereafter, two years of clinical work. The formation of the scientific medical doctor was in the process of being accomplished. The future of dedicated medical teachers and superior clinicians for the United States had been secured. Hopkins was making a unique contribution to the medical world!

Table 11.3. First Faculty of the Johns Hopkins Medical School established in 1893 in Baltimore, Maryland		
Name	Procedence	Area of Concentration
Clinical		
William Welch	New York	Pathology (and Medical School Dean)
Willliam Osler	Montreal	Medicine
William Halsted	New York	Surgery
Howard Kelly	Philadelphia	Obstetrics/Gynecology
Basic		
Franklin Pain Mall	Ann Arbor	Anatomy
John Jacob Abel	Ann Arbor	Pharmacology
William Howell	Ann Arbor	Physiology
Hospital Administrator		
Henry Hurd	Ann Arbor	Medical Administration

Conclusion

The formation of Johns Hopkins Medical School was a unique experiment in American medicine, a school that followed the German medical system in the basic sciences and British examples in clinical teaching. One to which a significant amount of American ingenuity was added. The Hopkins experiment would include, then, "a true center of learning and that its faculty would be made up of scholars capable of performing original research and of guiding graduate students along the path of creative scholarship" (Bordley and Harvey). With the commitment of dedicated professionals and an able administration, Hopkins scaled heights that had never been seen before. A unique group of individuals whose only incentive was to make good medicine and to improve its delivery and the science of it was represented by the Hopkins faculty. Medical education was their life and medical research was a way to open the doors of knowledge to society.

This extraordinary experiment would not have been completed if Mr. Hopkins had not endowed this university with the bequest already mentioned. The specifications of the will, the dedication of the trustees, faculty, and administration made this experiment succeed in an unimaginable way.

Some of the great names involved in this exceptional story would include: Johns Hopkins, Daniel Gilman, John Shaw Billings, William Welch, William Halsted, William Osler, Howard Kelly, Henry Hurd, Mary Garrett, Franklin Mall, John Abel, William Howell, and many others whose names remain untold such as the important board of trustees who were the engine behind this impressive model of medical education and health delivery.

CHAPTER 12
MODERN AMERICANS ARRIVE WITH MORE: THE TWENTIETH CENTURY UNFOLDS

As the twentieth century unfolded, Americans began to feel more comfortable about competing with Europeans, about demonstrating their ability to make medical discoveries, about their clinical knowledge, and about the maturity of their scientific background. In this section, we analyze only medical science at the closing of the nineteenth century and some of the most important discoveries of the first third of the twentieth century.

Closing of the Nineteenth Century

The nineteenth century had brought with it significant medical advances. Anesthesia (1846), the germ theory of the disease (1867), the better use of antiseptics, and the improved management of surgical disease were just some of the outstanding developments in which the nineteenth century based its unique record of progress and discovery. Physicians had turned the corner and began to accept science as the guiding principle of the practice of medicine of the times. Medicine began its better understanding of disease by seeking the origin of the pathology observed. Specific treatments were not all forthcoming since they required the accumulation of sufficient knowledge which was not existent at this particular time.

Of the important American medical advances attributed to the last quarter of the nineteenth century, one could consider the opening of important medical institutions such as the Hospital of the University of Michigan Medical School (1877), Michael Reese Hospital (1882), Johns Hopkins Hospital (1889), Mayo Clinic (1889), Johns Hopkins Medical School (1893), and several Hygienic Laboratories of Public Health. Next, we could describe the many bacteriological discoveries occurring in Europe and the United States. Because of our concentration in American medicine, we will only enumerate some of the American bacteriological advances such as the introduction of bacteriology in the United States by Welch, Prudden, Sternberg, and Salmon (1877) and the demonstration that killed bacterial cultures could be used as vaccines by Salmon and Smith (1886). Nuttall noted the antibacterial power of blood serum in the same year (1886), Sewall immunized pigeons against rattlesnake venom (1887), Sternberg opened the first private bacteriological laboratory in Brooklyn (1888), Welch discovered the bacillus of gas gangrene (1891), Sternberg first described viral neutralizing antibodies (1892), the same year Smith and Kilbourne demonstrated the tick-transmision of bovine piroplasmosis, and Gilbert discovered paracolon and paratyphoid bacilli (1893). As one can see, Americans were beginning to take active participation in the medical science most active of the day in Europe, bacteriology.

In the surgical sciences, there were important contributions by United States surgeons, particularly William Halsted of Hopkins. Halsted and his group introduced new surgical instruments (hemostat, 1878), a new way of conduction (regional) anesthesia (1885), the use of new techniques of bowel suture (1887), the use of rubber gloves (1889), new operations for inguinal hernia and cancer (1889), and the successful ligation of the first portion of the subclavian artery (1892). Conner performed a gastrectomy in Cincinnati (1883), Fitz described the pathology and clinical features of appendicitis (1886), McBurney presented the right lower quadrant as the area whose pain advised surgeons for the early operation for appendicitis (1889), and Brown catheterized the male ureter (1895).

Several outstanding medical societies began to be established (American Surgical Association (1880), Association of American Physicians (1886), American Orthopedic Association (1887), American Association of Anatomists (1888), Association of American Medical Colleges (1891), and others), various publications of recognized importance appeared (*Journal of the American Medical Association* (1883), *Journal of Experimental Medicine* (1896), and *American Journal of Physiology* (1898)), and the use of the new technique of X-ray (introduced in Germany by Roentgen in 1895) in this country by Cannon for the radiological visualization of the gastrointestinal tract (1896). Other discoveries occurred in late nineteenth century America, and of special mention is the incorporation of a new discipline, hormonal biochemistry, that grew of age when John Abel from Hopkins isolated and characterized epinephrine for the first time (1899). Bordley and Harvey gave us an excellent summary of the most significant discoveries and advances of American medicine of the latter part of the nineteenth century and a great deal of the twentieth century. We draw upon their findings for this overview of American contributions to modern medicine.

An Important Development: The Flexner Report

A unique and important perspective in American medicine was presented by the extraordinary report on medical education so timely advanced by Abraham Flexner (1866-1959) in 1910. His study on *Medical Education in the United States and Canada* was the pivotal document upon which reputable medical schools had to measure themselves to reach prominence and remain above the unique standards derived from this study. Flexner placed an ultimatum on all those schools that were failing the grade of maintaining American medical education at the highest scholarly standards of teaching and clinical practice.

The study of Flexner represented the most critical and important step to unraveling American medical education and to offer a new way to improve those medical schools that were not making the mark. He astutely divided the schools in various groups, those that were at the top—Hopkins, Michigan, Harvard, Pennsylvania, and others—which offered the best standards of medical education that the country could encounter up to that time; those at the bottom of the group that would require an enormous amount of work to reach the standards of excellence predicated by Flexner—many medical schools in this group could not be competitive enough and ended up closing their doors permanently—; and those schools in the middle of the pack that would need some support to remain viable.

The Flexner Report demanded an atmosphere of excellence in American medicine. Its standards became the ultimate goal for medicals around the country. Universities began to build upon the principles of this report and started to exert pressure on the medical schools under their jurisdiction. It was a matter of time before the whole country was regimented by the ideas and recommendations of this extraordinary document. The Flexner Report changed American medicine forever!

Early Twentieth Century: First Third

Americans had started their ascent to complete acceptance of scientific medicine. Their competition with Europeans would exert a fundamental effect in improving the practice of medicine in the world. Even though it wasn't until after World War II that American ingenuity surpassed Europeans in the science and technology of medicine, the first years of the twentieth century proved fruitful as well.

In the first third of the twentieth century (1900-1930), many American advances were incorporated into American medicine and the medicine of the world. Several noted medical institutions were founded such as the Rockefeller Institute for Medical Research (1901), the U.S. Public Health Service (1902), the Hospital of the Rockefeller Institute (1910), and Duke University Medical School (1930). Multiple medical discoveries occupied the attention of the American medical mind in the first decade (1900-1910); Solis-Cohn introduced the use of epinephrine for asthma (1900), Frazier sectioned the posterior (sensory) root of trigeminal nerve for neuralgia (1901), Young performed the first perineal prostatectomy (1902), Winter resuscitated the heart by injection with epinephrine (1905), Harrison introduced tissue culture (1907), Miles used a new operation for cancer of the rectum (1907), Cushing operated on the pituitary gland (1908), MacCallum and Voegtlin defined the relation of the parathyroids to calcium metabolism (1909), and Vedder identified the amebicidal effect of emetine (1910).

In the second decade of the century (1911-1920), Americans continued to bring innovative and practical discoveries to medical science as well as to develop new medical organizations oriented to foster better communication among the various specialty groups and at the same time to serve as a forum for the presentation of medical problems. In this regard, the American College of Surgeons (1913) and the American College of Physicians (1915) were founded. Years before, the American Society of Clinical Surgeons (1903), the American Genetic Association (1906), and the American Society for Clinical Investigation (1909) had already been incorporated.

The third decade of the twentieth century (1921-1930) was not different than the previous two decades. Americans did not stop at this stage, important works advanced in quality and quantity. The science of medicine had consistently grown, up to the point of being self sufficient and independent. Some highlights of this period were represented by works of Evans and Long who demonstrated the properties of the growth and gonadotropic hormones of the anterior pituitary gland (1921), McCollum and Steenbook discovered vitamin D (1922), Whipple observed the regenerative effect of the liver on experimental anemia in dogs (1922), Graham and Cole introduced oral cholecystography for the diagnosis of stone disease of the gallbladder (1923), Plummer recommended iodine therapy before surgery for Graves' disease (1923), Rowntree and Adson published the first sympathectomy for hypertension (1925), Minot and Murphy reported on the use of liver treatment for pernicious anemia, Goldberger isolated the pellagra-preventive factor, and Abel isolated insulin in crystalline form (all in 1926). Kennaway extracted the first known cancer-causing chemical 3, 4 benzpyrene (1926), Charles Mayo successfully removed a pheochromocytoma (1927), Churchill performed the first pericardiectomy for constrictive pericarditis in this country (1929), and a year later, Wilson, MacLeod, and Barker introduced the precordial lead for routine electrocardiograms (1930). The discovery of other vitamins which permitted the prevention of several deficiency diseases, the discovery of sulpha drugs, penicillin, and other antibiotics, which transformed the treatment of infections, and the introduction of diphtheria immunization are not part of this chapter since these events occurred later than our time period of the first third of the twentieth century.

Brief Remarks About the Rest of the Century

The American medical discoveries made in the first third of the twentieth century were just the beginning of a century that will be remembered as the most important in the annals of medical history. If the first third was significant, the second and third were even more prominent. American medical discoveries began to appear at a frequent pace and with a well-thought out scientific background. Cures for infectious diseases were very high in the list of accomplishments; the same was true for anti-neoplasic and anti-rejection drugs. Remarkable surgical procedures were introduced into clinical practice. Opening and repairing the heart, opening and tweaking the brain, replacing all kinds of organs, and substituting joints and limbs for artificial ones were some of the surgical feats of the twentieth century. Nothing was distant enough; medical scientists and clinicians successfully joined hands to overcome the medical problems of the time. There was no stop to unraveling important medical diseases.

The twentieth century had an enormous amount of discoveries derived from United States ingenuity. Many American medical and surgical discoveries alike were incorporated into clinical practice. From the benches of the laboratory to the patients' bedsides, new drugs, procedures, and ways of treatment were introduced and accepted by the medical profession. The twentieth century proved to be an oasis of American creativity and advanced medical care.

Notable developments in the medical sciences can be clearly traced to the twentieth century. In this century, immunology, cardiovascular diseases, neurological diseases, hematological problems, cancer, diabetes and endocrine diseases, among many in the medical field have been extensively studied and defined. Important and key advances were conquered in this century. The large number of Nobel awards in physiology and medicine bestowed upon American scientists and physicians attest to the high-caliber innovative work that they had accomplished during the last century. By design, it was not our intention in this section to discuss the incredible number of discoveries and advances realized by Americans in the last two thirds of the century. Our aim has been to provide a brief summary of the advances developed during the first third of the century, as a way to present the unfolding of this period of time as far as American ingenuity was concerned.

Conclusion

If nineteenth century medicine belonged to English, French, and German physicians and scientists, the twentieth century clearly belonged to American wisdom and ingenuity. In this century, the scientific character of American physicians reached an important pedestal among physicians of the world. Through systematic work, improved medical education, and research, Americans advanced in a significant fashion the medical knowledge of the day.

During the twentieth century, many discoveries began to occur on American soil. Americans educated in Europe in the second half of the nineteenth century or those educated in the United States, under strict scientific guidelines, introduced new findings in the new medicine of physiological or biochemical origin. Research became an American habit in many of the premier medical schools. Research, ingenuity, and dedicated work were the key factors in the extraordinary goals reached by American physicians and scientists of the time.

CHAPTER 13
CONCLUSIONS

American medical history possesses a long tradition of innovation and discovery. American Indians in the pre-colonial age offered specific remedies for the maladies of the times. English colonists did not have an improved system of medical care compared to the American Indian nations in early sixteenth century English America.

As time evolved, new European discoveries began to form a body of medical knowledge that would have a significant impact on the medicine of the world. Certainly, these findings needed a systematic approach and coordination. This would not happen until the late nineteenth century. In between, English medical America was slow in providing acceptable means of consistent medical support.

Formal education of the American physician in English America did not begin until the development of the first medical school in Philadelphia in 1765. The University of Pennsylvania Medical School organized its faculty following the system of the University of Edinburgh. Most of the initial Pennsylvania physicians had had a significant exposure to the Scottish university. Other medical schools followed through in the late eighteenth century, and in this way, Columbia, Harvard, and Dartmouth started.

In spite of the advances realized in medical education in English America, they were not sufficient to prepare the physicians of the epoch. The requirements placed on future physicians was limited in previous education (no bachelor's degree was required for admission) as well as the actual time spent in medical school (1 to 1½ years). It would not be until the last third of the nineteenth century that Harvard, Pennsylvania, and Michigan would considerably improve their standards to reach excellence in medical education. Then, in 1893, Hopkins would maximize medical education in this country and the rest of the world.

In 1809, an American physician, Ephraim McDowell, startled the world by removing an ovarian tumor of more than 100 pounds weight when anesthesia had not been formally established. In the 1820s, William Beaumont studied the gastric secretion in a patient with a gunshot wound to the stomach, and in the 1840s, Long, Morton, Wells, and Jackson introduced the use of ether for surgical anesthesia. These discoveries did not change the American mind which still remained pragmatic as far as science was concerned.

The American Civil War presented another opportunity for medical advances, particularly in the care of the wounded soldier: amputations, blood vessel ligations, the use of anesthesia, plastic procedures of the face, transportation of the wounded, and many other advances were apparent at the end of this sanguineous event. Both sides, the Confederate and the Union, had to establish a medical system that would permit the care of thousands of soldiers suffering the effects of the battlefield as well as that of the diseases of the day, particularly those associated with the infectious diseases so prevalent at the time. At the end of the Civil War hostilities, physicians had gained more experience in the management of multiple pathologies as well as in the treatment of massive casualties secondary to battlefield injuries.

When the nineteenth century began closing, in the 1890s, medical education and scientific discovery had started an ascending path. Physicians were more aware of the importance of innovation and research. Some medical schools were offering improved curriculum, and in 1893, the Hopkins medical school system presented the best example of high level medical education in the nation. Education, research, and discovery were now beginning to speak the same language, one of necessity, importance, and academic leadership.

The twentieth century constituted a unique example for the maximal development of medicine in the United States of America. Physicians, scientists, and educators participated in a common goal of reaching out to the best in medical care, the best in teaching and medical education, and the best in research and discovery. As the first third of the twentieth century started its expansion, medicine began to reach heights that had never been obtained before. American medicine was ready to establish an individual mark that would characterize its future development, was continuing its accelerating growth, and was aware of its responsibility in the medicine of the world. It is not surprising that when the second half of the twentieth century appeared, Americans were contributing in every field possible to medical science and practice. American medicine was here to stay, and Americans were ready to sustain its dedicated and committed progress.

BIBLIOGRAPHY

Preface

Cassedy JH. *Medicine in America. A Short History*. Baltimore, MD: Johns Hopkins University Press; 1991.

Duffy J. *The Healers: A History of American Medicine*. Urbana, IL: University of Illinois Press; 1979.

Packard FR. *A History of Medicine in the United States*. Vol. I and II. New York: Hafner Publishing Company; 1963.

Chapter 1: Europeans Invade Indian America

Blanton WB. *Medicine in Virginia in the Seventeenth Century*. Richmond, Virginia: The William Byrd Press Inc.; 1930.

Burke JG. *Apache Medicine-Men*. New York: Dover Publications; 1993

Catton B, Catton WB. *The Bold and Magnificent Dream: America's Founding Years, 1492-1815*. Garden City: Doubleday and Company, Inc.; 1978.

Duffy J. *The Healers: A History of American Medicine*. Urbana, Illinois: University Illinois Press; 1979.

Duffy J. Medicine and Medical Practices Among Aboriginal American Indians. In: Marti-Ibanez F, ed. *History of American Medicine*. New York: MD Publications, Inc.; 1958.

Dunlap MJ. Early American Rum Trade Proved Deadly Medicine. American Indians. 11 July 1995. Available at: http://www.ur.ku.edu/News/95N/JulyNews/July11/rumtrade.html

Garland J. *The Story of Medicine*. Boston: Houghton Mifflin Company; 1949.

Gordon MB. *Aesculapius Comes to the Colonies*. New Jersey: Ventnor Publishers; 1949.

Guthrie D. *A History of Medicine*. Philadelphia: J.B. Lippencott Company; 1946.

Hamerschlag CA. *The Dancing Healers*. New York: Harper Collins Publishers; 1988.

Hand WD. *American Folk Medicine: A Symposium*. Los Angeles: University of California Press; 1976.

Kupperman KO. *Settling with the Indians: The Meeting of English and Indian Cultures in America, 1580-1640*. New Jersey: Rowman and Littlefield; 1980.

Moerman DE. *Medicinal Plants of Native America*. Ann Arbor: University of Michigan Museum of Anthropology; 1986.

Morgan T. *Wilderness at Dawn: The Settling of the North American Continent.* New York: Simon and Schuster; 1993.

Quinn A. *A New World: An Epic of Colonial America from the Founding of Jamestown to the Fall of Quebec.* Boston: Faber and Faber; 1994.

Reiss O. *Medicine in Colonial America.* Lanham, Maryland: University Press of America; 2000.

Rosenberg CE. The Book in the Sickroom: A Tradition of Print and Practice. Available at: http://www.librarycompany.org/doctor/rosen.html#tennentb

Rothstein WG. *American Physicians in the Nineteenth Century.* Baltimore: Johns Hopkins University; 1972.

Shryock RH. *Medicine In America: Historical Essays.* Baltimore: Johns Hopkins University; 1966.

Siegel-Maier K. The Native Spirit. 28 July 1998. Available at: http://www.suite101.com/article.cfm/botanical_retired/8768

Siegel-Maier K. The Native Spirit II. 4 Aug. 1998. Available at: http://www.suite101.com/article.cfm/botanical_retired/8769.

Stone E. *Medicine Among the American Indians.* New York: Hafner Publishing Company; 1962.

Toledo-Pereyra LH. Origins of Surgery in British Colonial America. *J Invest Surg.* 2003; 16:3.

Trenton P, Houlihan PT. *Native Americans: Five Centuries of Changing Images.* New York: Harry N. Abrams Inc.; 1989.

Vogel VJ. *American Indian Medicine.* Norman: University of Oklahoma Press; 1970.

Chapter 2: Colonists Impose Themselves

Beck JB. *Medicine in the American Colonies.* New York: Horn & Wallace Publishers; 1850.

Bell JB. *The Colonial Physician.* New York: Science History Publications; 1975.

Blanton WB. *Medicine in Virginia in the Eighteenth Century.* Richmond: Garrett & Massie, Inc.; 1931.

Boorstein DJ. *The Americans: The Colonial Experience.* New York: Vintage Books; 1958.

Christianson EH. Medicine in New England. In: Leavitt JW, Numbers RL, eds. *Readings in Health in America.* Madison, WI: University of Wisconsin Press; 1997.

Doctors of medicine profession. Available at: http://www.nlm.nih.gov/medlineplus/ency/article/001936.htm.

Duffy J. *The Healers: A History of American Medicine.* Urbana, IL: University Illinois Press; 1979.

Finger S. *Doctor Franklin's Medicine.* Philadelphia, PA: University of Pennsylvania Press; 2006.

Frienenberg ZB. *The Doctor in Colonial America.* Danbury, CT: Rutledge Books; 1998.

Garrison FH. *History of Medicine.* Philadelphia: W.B. Saunders Company; 1929.

Gilder C. Childbirth in early America. Available at: http://www.gliah.uh.edu/historyonline/childbirth.cfm.

Gordon MB. *Aesculapius Comes to the Colonies*. New York: Argosy-Antiquarian, Ltd.; 1949.

Greeley J, Wilkinson S. Travel, Yes – Vacation, No: Crossing the Atlantic In Colonial Times. *River Gazette*. September 2003; page 6. Available at: http://www.smcm.edu/rivergazette/articles/03-3-5-6.pdf (River Gazette Article)

Gwilt JR, Gwilt PR. Native American medicines. *The Pharmaceutical Journal*. December 23, 2000; 265:940-941.

Haggard HW. *The Doctor in History*. New Haven: Yale University Press; 1934.

Major RH. *A History of Medicine*. Illinois: Bannerstone House; 1954.

Martha Ballard's Diary Online. Available at: www.dohistory.org

McGrew RE, McGrew MP. *Encyclopedia of Medical History*. New York: McGraw-Hill Book Company; 1985.

Reiss O. *Medicine in Colonial America*. Maryland: University Press of America; 2000.

Religion, education, and medicine in colonial America. Available at: http://www.usahistory.info/colonial/education.html.

Shryock RH. *Medicine and Society in America*. New York: New York University Press; 1960.

Silverman K. *Life and Times of Cotton Mather*. New York: Harpert & Row Publishers; 1984.

Smallpox. Available at: www.smplanet.com/colonial/disease/mather.html.

Smallpox: Cotton Mather, Minister of Inoculation. Available ate: http://www.smplanet.com/colonial/disease/mather.html.

Stenn F. *The Growth of Medicine*. Illinois: Bannerstone House; 1967.

Toledo-Pereyra LH. First American Medical Schools. In *Vignettes on Surgery, History and Humanities*. Toledo-Pereyra LH, ed. Georgetown, TX: Landes Bioscience; 2005.

Ulrich LT. *Good Wives: Image and Reality in the Lives of Women in Northern New England, 1650-1750*. New York: Vintage Books; 1991.

Chapter 3: Europeans Knew Medicine Before

Bass JH. *The History of Medicine and the Medical Profession*. Huntington: Robert E. Krieger Publishing Co. Inc.; 1971.

Blanton WB. *Medicine in Virginia in the Seventeenth Century*. Richmond, Virginia: The William Byrd Press Inc.; 1930.

Debus AG., ed. *Medicine in Seventeenth Century England*. Berkley, CA: University of California Press; 1974.

Doig A, Ferguson JPS, Milne IA, and Passmore R. *William Cullen and the Eighteenth Century Medical World*. Edinburgh: Edinburgh University Press; 1993.

Duffy J. *The Healers: A History of American Medicine*. Urbana, IL: University Illinois Press; 1979.

Harvey W. *An Anatomical Disputation Concerning the Movement of the Heart and Blood in Living Creatures*. Whitteridge G transl. Oxford: Blackwell Scientific; 1976.

Gregory A. *Harvey's Heart: The Discovery of Blood Circulation*. Cambridge, England: Icon Books Ltd.; 2001.

Keele K. *William Harvey: The Man, the Physician, and the Scientist*. London: Nelson; 1965.

Keynes G. *The Life of William Harvey*. Oxford: Clarendon Press; 1978.

Lindeboom GA. *Herman Boerhaave: The Man and His Work*. London: Methuen & Co. Ltd.; 1968.

Moore W. *The Knife Man: The Extraordinary Life and Times of John Hunter, Father of Modern Surgery*. New York: Broadway Books; 2005.

Porter R. *The Greatest Benefit to Mankind: A Medical History of Humanity*. New York: W. W. Norton and Co.; 1997.

Reiss O. *Medicine in Colonial America*. Maryland: University Press of America; 2000.

Robinson V. *The Story of Medicine*. New York: Tudor Publishing Co.; 1931.

Sigerist HE. *The Great Doctors: A Biographical History of Medicine*. Freeport, NY: Books for Libraries Press; reprinted 1971.

Sigerist HE. *Henry E. Sigerist on the History of Medicine*. New York: MD Publications; 1960.

Sigerist HE. *A History of Medicine Vol. I: Primitive and Archaic Medicine*. New York: Oxford University Press; 1955.

Simmons JG. *Doctors and Discoveries: Lives that Created Today's Medicine*. New York: Houghton Mifflin Company; 2002.

Singer C, Underwood EA. *A Short History of Medicine*. 2nd ed. New York: Oxford University Press; 1962.

Talbott JH. *A Biographical History of Medicine*. New York: Grune and Stratton, Inc.; 1970.

Toledo-Pereyra LH, ed. *Vignettes on Surgery, History and Humanities*. Georgetown, TX: Landes Bioscience; 2005.

Underwood EA. *Boerhaave's Men*. Edinburgh: Edinburgh University Press; 1977.

Venzmer G. *Five Thousand Years of Medicine*. New York: Taplinger; 1968.

Wear A. *Knowledge and Practice in English Medicine, 1550-1680*. New York: Cambridge University Press; 2000.

Chapter 4: Medicine Gets Academic

Beecher HK, Altschule MD. *Medicine at Harvard: The First Three Hundred Years*. Hanover, New Hampshire: University Press of New England; 1977.

Black T. History of the Deans–Part I of III, 1850-1891. Medicine at Michigan. 2001. Available at: http://www.medicineatmichigan.org/magazine/1999/fall/deanhistory/default.asp

Bramucci N. Institutionalization of Medical Education. Medical Care In The City of Baltimore 1752-1919. October 2, 2003. Available at: http://www.mdhistoryonline.net/mdmedicine/cfm/pt2.cfm

Castiglioni A. *A History of Medicine*. 2nd ed. Translated by E.B. Krumbhaar, MD, Ph.D. New York: Alfred A. Knopf; 1947.

Chapman CB. *Dartmouth Medical School: The First 175 Years*. Hanover: University Press of New England; 1973.

Cheyney EP. *History of the University of Pennsylvania 1740-1940*. Philadelphia: University of Philadelphia Press; 1940.

Corner GW. *Two Centuries of Medicine: A History of the School of Medicine, University of Pennsylvania*. Philadelphia: J.B. Lippincott Company; 1965.

Davenport HW. *Fifty Years of Medicine at The University of Michigan: 1891-1941*. Ann Arbor: University of Michigan Medical School; 1986.

Duffy J. *Epidemics in Colonial America*. Baton Rouge: Louisiana State University Press; 1971.

Duffy J. *From Humors to Medical Science: A History of American Medicine*. 2nd ed. Urbana: University of Illinois Press; 1993.

Gill HB. *The Apothecary in Colonial Virginia*. Charlottesville: University Press of Virginia; 1972.

A History of Columbia University 1754-1904. New York: Columbia University Press; 1904.

History of the School of Medicine. University Archives and Records Center, University of Pennsylvania. Available at: http://www.archives.upenn.edu/histy/schools/med.html

HMS History. Available at: www.hms.harvard.edu/about/history.html

Humphrey DC. *From King's College to Columbia 1746-1800*. New York: Columbia University Press; 1976.

Kelley BM. *Yale: A History*. New Haven: Yale University Press; 1974.

Leavitt JW, Numbers RL, eds. *Sickness and Health in America: Readings in the History of Medicine and Public Health*. 3rd ed. Madison: University of Wisconsin Press; 1997.

Luft E. The Earliest North American Medical Schools: Chronological List of Founding Dates. State University of New York Upstate Medical University Health Sciences Library. 2003. Available at: http://www.upstate.edu/library/history/medschoolfoundingdates.html

Medicine at Yale, 1701-1901. Available at: http://info.med.yale.edu/library/exhibits/yalemed1/medinstyalecoll.html

Rothstein WG. *American Medical Schools and the Practice of Medicine: A History*. New York: Oxford University Press; 1987.

Shryock RH. *The Unique Influence of the Johns Hopkins University on American Medicine*. Copenhagen: Ejnar Munksgaard, Ltd.; 1953.

Singer C, Underwood AE. *A Short History of Medicine*. London: Oxford University Press; 1962.

Toledo AH. The Medical Legacy of Benjamin Rush. *Journal of Investigative Surgery*. 17:61-63; 2004.

Toledo-Pereyra LH, ed. *Vignettes on Surgery, History and Humanities*. Georgetown, TX: Landes Bioscience; 2005.
University of Maryland School of Medicine. September 2002. Available at: http://medschool.umaryland.edu/newabout.asp

Chapter 5: And Now We Can Put Them to Sleep

Agony!: From Agony to Anesthesia. JLR Medical Group. 2002. Available at: http://www.jlrmedicalgroup.com/agony.htm
Angle G, Harding RS. Crawford W. Long Collection, 1842-1926, #120. Available at Http://americanhistory.si.edu/archives/d9120/htm
Bollet AJ. *Civil War Medicine: Challenges and Triumphs*. Tucson, AZ: Galen Press, Ltd.; 2002
Clarke E. *Modern Methods in the History of Medicine*. London: Athlone Press of the University of London; 1971.
Doyle SR. Anesthetic Agents: Inhaled Anesthetics. October 18, 2000. Available at: Http://www.nurse-anesthesia.com/inhaledanesthetics.htm
Duffy J. *From Humors to Medical Science*. 2nd ed. Champaign, IL: University of Illinois; 1993.
Evans T. The Unusual History of Ether. Anesthesia Nursing and Medicine. 2003. Available at: http://www.anesthesia-nursing.com/ether.html
Fenster JM. *Ether Day*. New York: Perennial Harper Collins; 2001.
Fradin DB. *We have Conquered Pain: the Discovery of Anesthesia*. New York: Margaret K. McElderry Books; 1996.
Friedman G, Friedman M. *Medicine's 10 Greatest Discoveries*. New Haven, CT: Yale University Press; 1998.
Gordon R. *The Alarming History of Pain: Amusing Anecdotes from Hippocrates to Heart Transplants*. New York: St. Martin's Press; 1993.
History of Anesthesia. Anesthesia Today. 1999. Available at: http://204.178.120.164/history.asp
Medicine's greatest gift. Neurosurgical Service, Massachusetts General Hospital and Harvard University. 2000. Available at: Http://neurosurgery.mgh.harvard.edu/History/gift.htm
Nuland SB. *The Origins of* Anesthesia. Birmingham, AL: The Classics of Medicine Library; 1983.
Simmons JG. *Doctors & Discoveries: Lives that created Today's Medicine, from Hippocrates to the present*. Boston: Houghton Mifflin Company; 2002
Toledo-Pereyra LH, ed. *Vignettes on Surgery, History and Humanities*. Georgetown, TX: Landes Bioscience; 2005.
Vertosick FT. *Why we Hurt: The Natural History of Pain*. Sherman Oaks, CA: Hartcourt Inc.; 2000.
Welty G. The Emergence of the Modern Mode of Medical Production. *Humanity and Society*. November 1985.

Chapter 6: Not Only Regular Doctors Cure

Barret S. Notes on Homeopathy's History. Alternative Medicine: A Skeptical

Look. Available at: http://www.canoe.ca/HealthAlternativeColumns/011206.html

Binger C. *Revolutionary Doctor: Benjamin Rush.* New York: W.W. Norton and Company; 1966.

Bollett AJ. *Civil War Medicine: Triumphs and Challenges.* Tucson, AZ: Galen Press, Ltd.; 2002.

Booth ER. *History of Osteopathy and Twentieth-Centure Medical Practice.* Cincinnati: Caxton Press; 1924.

Cooter R. *Phrenology in the British Isles.* Metuchen, NJ: Scarecrow Press, Inc.; 1989.

Duffy J. *The Healers: A History of American Medicine.* Urbana IL: University of Illinois Press; 1976.

Ernst W. *Plural Medicine, Tradition, and Modernity, 1800-2000.* New York: Rutledge, Taylor, and Francis Group; 2002.

Floyd B. Scientific Medicine. University of Toledo Libraries. Available at: http://www.cl.utoledo.edu/canaday/quackery/quack2.html

Gevtiz N. *Other Healers: Unorthodox Medicine in America.* Baltimore, MD: Johns Hopkins University Press; 1988.

Green CG, Stone M, Theo T. *The Transformation of Psychology.* Washington, DC: American Psychological Association; 2001.

Halter JS. *The People's Doctor.* Carbondale, IL: Southern Illinois University Press; 1992.

Kaufman M. *Homeopathy in America.* Baltimore, MD: John Hopkins Press; 1971.

Kett, JF. *The Formation of the American Medical Profession.* New Haven, CT: Yale University Press; 1968.

Numbers RL. The Fall and Rise of the American Medical Profession in Leavitt JW, Numbers RL. *Sickness and Health in America.* Madison, WI: The University of Wisconsin Press; 1985.

Packard FR. *History of Medicine in the United States.* Vol. II. New York: Hafner Publishing Company; 1963.

Rothstein WJ. *American Physicians in the Nineteenth Century.* Baltimore, MD: Johns Hopkins University Press; 1971.

Schoepflin RB. Christian Science Healing in America in Gevtiz N. *Other Healers: Unorthodox Medicine in America.* Baltimore, MD: Johns Hopkins University Press; 1988.

Simmons JG. *Doctors and Discoveries.* Boston, MA: Houghton Mifflin Company; 2002.

Steele V. *Bleed, Blister, and Purge: A History of Medicine on the American Frontier.* Missoula, MT: Mountain Press Publ. Co.; 2005.

Van Wyhe J. The History of Phrenology on the Web. 2002. Available at: http://pages.britishlibrary.net/phrenology/overview.htm

Walsh J. Medicine at Michigan State. Parts I, II, III, and IV. *Science.* 177:1085, 1972; 178:136, 1972; 178:288, 1972; and 177:377, 1972.

Wardwell WI. Chiropractors: Evolution to Acceptance in Gevtiz N. *Other Healers: Unorthodox Medicine in America.* Baltimore, MD: Johns

Hopkins University Press; 1988.
Worthen JC. *Nature Cures: The History of Alternative Medicine in America.* New York: Oxford University Press; 2002.
Wroebel A. *Pseudo Science and Society in nineteenth Century America.* Lexington: University of Kentucky; 1987.

Chapter 7: Not for White Men Only

Bonner TN. *To the Ends of the Earth: Women's Search for Education in Medicine.* Cambridge, MA: Harvard University Press; 1985.
Brandt AM. Racism and Research in Leavitt JW and Numbers RL, eds., *Sickness and Health in America*, 2d. ed. Madison, WI: University of Wisconsin Press; 1985.
Chaff SL. *Women in Medicine: A Bibliography of the Literature on Women Physicians.* Metuchen, NJ: Scarecrow Press; 1977.
Drachman V. *Hospital with a Heart: Women Doctors and the Paradox of Separatism at the New England Hospital, 1862-1969.* Ithaca, NY: Cornell University Press; 1984.
Dyson W. *Howard University: The Capstone of Negro Education, A History 1867-1940.* Washington, DC: The Graduate School Howard University; 1941.
Gordon RC. Charles R. Drew: Surgeon, Scientist, and Educator. *Journal of Investigative Surgery.* 18:223-225; 2005.
-------- Daniel Hale Williams: Pioneer Black Surgeon and Educator. *Journal of Investigative Surgery.* 18:105-106; 2005.
Hayden RC. *11 African American Doctors.* Frederick, MD: Twenty-First Century Books; 1992.
Hornsby Jr. A. Black Americans in *The World Book Encyclopedia.* Chicago: World Book, Inc.; 1985, p. 306.
Jacobi MP. Women in Medicine in Meyer AN, ed., *Woman's Work in America.* New York: 1891.
Kent D. *Elizabeth Blackwell: Physician and Health Educator.* Chanhassen, MN: The Child's World Editors; 2004.
Matthew S. *The First Woman of Medicine: The Story of Elizabeth Blackwell.* New York: Contemporary Perspectives, Inc.; 1978.
May ET. *Young Oxford History of Women in the United States.* New York: Oxford University Press; 1993.
Morais HM. *The History of the Negro in Medicine.* New York: Publishers Company Inc.; 1967
Morantz RM. The Connecting Link: The Case for the Woman Doctor in 19th Century America in Leavitt JW and Numbers RL, eds., *Sickness and Health in America*, 2d. ed. Madison, WI: University of Wisconsin Press; 1985.
Morantz-Sanchez R. *Sympathy and Science.* New York: Oxford University Press; 1985.
Numbers RL, Savitt TL. *Science and Medicine in the Old South.* Baton Rouge,

LA: Louisiana State University Press; 1989.

First 3 African American physicians. Accessed July 18, 2006. Available at http://ohoh.essortment.com/africanamerican_rqdo.htm

Peitzman SJ. *A New and Untried Course: Women's Medical College and Medical College of Pennsylvania, 1850-1998*. New Brunswick, NJ: Rutgers University Press; 2000.

Savitt TL. *Medicine and Slavery: The Diseases and Healthcare of Blacks in Antebellum Virginia*. Urbana, IL: University of Illinois Press; 1978.

---------Black Health on the Plantation in Leavitt JW and Numbers RL, eds., *Sickness and Health in America*, 2d. ed. Madison, WI: University of Wisconsin Press; 1985a.

---------Lincoln University Medical Department: A Forgotten 19th Century Black Medical School. *J Hist Med Allied Sciences*. 40:42-65; 1985b.

Stille DR. *Extraordinary Women of Medicine*. New York: Children Press, Grolier Publishing; 1997.

Summerville J. *Educating Black Doctors: A History of Meharry Medical College*. Birmingham, AL: The University of Alabama Press; 1983.

Toledo-Pereyra LH, ed. *Vignettes on Surgery, History and Humanities*. Georgetown, TX: Landes Bioscience; 2005.

www.danielwilliams.html

Chapter 8: Nation up in Arms

Adams GW. *Doctors in Blue: The Medical History of the Union Army in the Civil War*. New York: Henry Shuman; 1952.

Barnes JK. *The Medical and Surgical History of the War of Rebellion (1861-1865)*. Washington, DC: Gov. Printing Office, 1870-1888.

Beller SP. *Medical Practices in the Civil War*. Cincinnati, OH: Betterway Books; 1992.

Bollett AJ. *Civil War Medicine: Challenges and Triumphs*. Tucson, AZ: Galen Press; 2002.

-------- All those Amputations. *Resident and Staff Physician*. 1999; 45:83-85.

Cassedy JH. *Medicine in America: A Short History*. Baltimore, MD: The Johns Hopkins University Press; 1991.

Catton B. *The American Heritage Picture History of the Civil War*. New York: American Heritage Pub. Co.; 1960.

Chisolm JJ. *A Manual of Military Surgery for the Use of Surgeons in the Confederate Army*. 3d ed. Columbia, SC: Evans & Cogswell; 1864.

Civil War Medicine. Available at: eHistory.com.

Cunningham HH. *Doctors in Gray: The Confederate Medical Service*. Baton Rouge, LA: Louisiana State University Press; 1958.

Dammann G. *Pictorial Encyclopedia of Civil War Medical Instruments and Equipment*. Missoula, MT: Pictorial Histories Publishing Company; 1983.

Duncan LC. *The Medical Department of the United States Army in the Civil War*. Gaithersburg, MD: Butternut Press; 1985

Freemon FR. *Gangrene and Glory: Medical Care During the American Civil War*. Cranbury, NJ: Fairleigh Dickinson University Press; 1998.

Gordon JB. *Reminiscences of the Civil War*. New York: C. Scribner's Sons; 1905.

Hart AG. *The Surgeon and the Hospital in the Civil War*. Gaithersburg, MD: Olde Soldier Books; 1987

The History Place. 2003. Available at: www.historyplace.com

Key JD. The U.S. Army Medical Department in the Civil War. *Mil Med* 1968; 133:185-186.

McPherson J. *Battle Cry of Freedom: The Civil War Era*. Oxford, England: Oxford University Press; 1988.

Mitchell SW. On the Medical Department in the Civil War. *JAMA* 1914; 62:1445-1450.

National Museum of Civil War Medicine. Available at: www.civilwarmed.org

Pember PY. *A Southern Woman's Story: Life in Confederate Richmond.* Bell Irvin Wiley, ed. Jackson, TN: 1959.

Rutkow I. *Bleeding Blue and Gray*. New York: Random House Publishers; 2005.

Schroeder-Lein GR. *Confederate Hospitals on the Move: Samuel H. Stout and the Army of Tennessee*. Columbia, SC: University of South Carolina Press; 1994.

Shultz SM, Casady RL, Hoffman RR, Flowers BK, Fielding LP. The Last Confederate Casualty at Gettysburg: A Case Report and Review of Similar Historic Cases. *J. Amer. Coll. Surg.* 2000; 191:204-207.

Stillé CJ. *History of the United States Sanitary Commission*. New York: Hurd and Houghton; 1868.

Toledo-Pereyra LH, Toledo AH. American Civil War. Part II. *Journal of Investigative Surgery*. 17:115-117; 2004.

-------- American Civil War. Part II. *Journal of Investigative Surgery*. 17:185-189; 2004.

Chapter 9: Americans Reject Science

Ackerknecht EH. The Fielding H. Garrison Lecture: Anticontagionism Between 1821 and 1867. *Bull His Med.* 1948; 22:562.

Bonner TA. *Becoming a Physician: Medical Education in Britain, France, Germany, and the United States, 1740-1945*. New York: Oxford University Press; 1995.

Bordley J, Harvey AM. *Two Centuries of American Medicine*. Philadelphia: W. B. Saunders, Co.; 1976.

Bruce RV. *The Launching of Modern American Science 1846-1876*. Ithaca, NY: Cornell Univ. Press; 1987

Bynum WF. *Science and the Practice of Medicine in the Nineteenth Century*. Cambridge, England: Cambridge Univ. Press; 1994.

Camp J. *The Healer's Art: The Doctor Through History*. New York: Taplinger Publishing Co; 1977.

Clendening L. *Source Book of Medical History*. New York: Dover Publications Inc.; 1942
De Baz P. *The Story of Medicine*. New York: Philosophical Library; 1975.
Doolin W. *Wayfarers In Medicine*. London: William Heinemann Medical Books Ltd; 1949.
Duffy J. *The Healers: A History of American Medicine*. Urbana, IL: Univ. Illinois Press; 1976.
Flexner A. *Medical Education in the United States and Canada. A Report to the Carnegie Foundation for the Advancement of Teaching*. New York: Arno Press; 1972 (originally published in 1910).
Inglis B. *A History of Medicine*. Cleveland: World Publishing Company; 1965.
Leavitt JW, Numbers RL. *Sickness and Health in America*. Madison, WI: The University of Wisconsin Press; 1985.
Louis Pasteur (1822-1895). Access Excellence @ the National Health Museum. 1999. Available at: www.accessexcellence.org/AB/BC/Louis_Pasteur.html
Ludmerer KM. *Time to Heal: American Medical Education from the Turn of the Century to the Era of Managed Care*. Oxford: Oxford University Press; 1999.
McGrew RE, McGrew M. *Encyclopedia of Medical History.* New York: McGraw-Hill Book Comp; 1985.
Miller G. One Hundred Years Ago. *Bull Hist Med.* 1947; 21:488.
Rothstein WG. *American Physicians in the Nineteenth Century.* Baltimore: Johns Hopkins Univ Press; 1972.
Simmons JG. *Doctors and Discoveries: Lives That Created Today's Medicine*. Boston: Houghton Mifflin Comp; 2002.
Stevenson LG. Science Down The Drain: On the Hostility of Certain Sanitarians to Animal Experimentation, Bacteriology, and Immunology. *Bull His Med.* 1955; 29:1.
Toledo-Pereyra LH, Toledo MM. Anticontagionism in the Opposition to Lister. *Current Surgery.* 1979; 39:78.
-------- A Critical Study of Lister's Work on Antiseptic Surgery. *Amer J Surg.* 1976; 131:736.
Tomes NJ. American Attitudes Toward the Germ Theory of the Disease: Phyllis Allen Richmond Revisited. *J Hist Allied Sc.* 1997; 52:7-16.
Virchow R. Standpoints in Scientific Medicine. In: Rather LJ, ed. *Disease, Life and Man: Selected Essays by Rudolf Virchow*. Stanford, CA: 1958:31.
Welch WH. Some of the Conditions Which Have Influenced the Development of American Medicine, Especially During the Last Century. *Bull Johns Hopkins Hosp.* 1908; 19:33.

Chapter 10: Knife at Work and the Bugs What

Ackerknecth EH. Anticontagionism Between 1821 and 1867. *Bull Hist Med.* 22:562-593.
-------- *A Short History of Medicine.* New York: Ronald Press Company; 1968.

Agnew DH. *The Principles and Practice of Surgery*. Vol. 1. Philadelphia: JB Lippincott; 1878.

Asepsis and Antisepsis. Surgical-tutor.org.uk. 2002. Available at: http://www.surgical-tutor.org.uk/core/preop1/asepsis.htm

Blanton WB. *Medicine in Virginia in the Eighteenth Century*. Richmond: Garrett & Massie, Inc.; 1931.

-------- *Medicine in Virginia in the Nineteenth Century*. Richmond: Garrett & Massie, Inc.; 1933.

A Brief History of Infectious Disease. Bayer Pharmaceutical Division, North America. 2002. Available at: http://www.bayerpharma-na.com/healthcare/hc0108.asp

Cameron HC. *Reminiscence of Lister*. Glasgow: Jackson, Eylie & Co; 1927.

Earl AS. *Surgery in America*. 2nd Ed. New York: Praeger Publishers; 1983.

Evans T. The Unusual History of Ether. Anesthesia Nursing and Medicine. 2003. Available at: http://www.anesthesia-nursing.com/ether.html

Fatout P. *Letters of a Civil War Surgeon*. West Lafayette, IN: Purdue University Studies; 1961.

Friedmand M, Friedland GW. *Medicine's 10 Greatest Discoveries*. New Haven: Yale University Press; 1998.

The germ theory of disease. Timelinescience resources. 2002. Available at: http://www.timelinescience.org/resource/students/pencilin/germ_th.htm

Green JR. *Medical History for Students*. Springfield, IL: Charles C. Thomas; 1968.

Gross SD. *A System of Surgery: Pathological, Diagnostic, Therapeutic, and Operative*. 5th ed. Philadelphia; 1872.

Joseph Lister (1827-1912). Surgical-tutor.org.uk. 2003. Available at: http://www.surgical-tutor.org.uk/default-home.htm?surgeons/lister.htm~right

Lister Centenary Exhibition at the Wellcome Historical Medical Museum. London: Wellcome Foundation Ltd.; 1927.

Lister J. Antiseptic Principle of the Practice of Surgery, 1867. In: Halsall P, ed. *Modern History Sourcebook: Joseph Lister (1827-1912)*. 1998. Available at: http://www.fordham.edu/halsall/mod/1867lister.html

-------- *Collected Papers*. 2nd vol. Oxford: Clarendon; 1909.

Loudon I. *The Oxford Ilustrated History of Western Medicine*. New York: Oxford University Press; 1997.

Lynn J. *Confederate Commando and Fleet Surgeon*. Shippensburg, PA: Burd Street Press; 2001.

The Norton Anthology of American Literature. 5th ed. Vol. 1. New York: W.W. Norton & Company, Inc.; 1998.

Nuland S. *Doctors: The Biography of Medicine*. New York: Vintage Books; 1989.

Richmond PA. American Attitudes Towards the Germ Theory of Disease (1860-1880). *J Hist Med & All Sciences*. 1954; 9:428-454.

Robinson V. *The Story of Medicine*. New York: Tudor Publishing Company;

1931.

Rothstein WG. *American Physicians in the Nineteenth Century*. Baltimore: Johns Hopkins Univ. Press; 1972.

Rutkow IM. *American Surgery: An Illustrated History*. Philadelphia: Lippincott-Raven Publishers; 1998.

-------- *Surgery: An Illustrated History*. St. Louis, MO: Mosby-Yearbook; 1993.

-------- Zabdiel Boylston and the Earliest Published Account of an Elective Surgical Operation in Colonial America. Arch Surg [serial online]. February 2002; 137:227. Available at: http://archsurg.ama-assn.org/content/vol137/issue2/index.dtl

Sigerist HE. Surgery at the time of the introduction of antisepsis. *J Missouri Med Assoc*. 1935; 32:174.

Simmons JG. *Doctors and Discoveries: Lives That Created Today's Medicine*. Boston: Houghton Mifflin Company; 2002.

Toledo-Pereyra LH, Toledo MM. Anticontagionism in the Opposition to Lister. *Current Surgery*. 1979; 39:78.

-------- *Maestros de la Cirugia Contemporanea*. Mexico: Ed. Ciencia y Cultura Latinoamericana; 1999.

-------- *Maestros de la Cirugia Moderna*. Mexico: Ed. Fondo de Cultura Economica; 1996.

-------- Our Surgical Heritage: A Critical Study of Lister's Work on Antiseptic Surgery. *Amer J Surg*. 1976:736-744.

-------- *Vignettes on Surgery, History and Humanities*. Georgetown, TX: Landes Bioscience; 2005.

Tomes NJ. American Attitudes Toward the Germ Theory of the Disease: Phyllis Allen Richmond Revisited. *J Hist Med Allied Sci*. 1997; 52:7-16.

Wangensteen OH. Nineteenth century wound management of the parturient uterus and compound fractures: the Semelweis-Lister Priority Controversy. *Bull NY Acad Sci*. 1970; 46:577.

Warren JC. *To Work in the Vineyard of Surgery*. Ed. Edward D. Churchill. Cambridge, Mass: Harvard University Press; 1958.

Watson BA. Disease germs; their origin, nature and relation to wounds. *Am Med Assoc Trans*. 1878; 2:281.

Williams G. *The Age of Miracles*. Chicago: Academy Chicago Publishers; 1987.

Zimmerman L, Veith I. *Great Ideas in the History of Surgery*. New York: Dover Publications, Inc.; 1967.

Chapter 11: Hopkins Takes the Lead

Billings JS. A review of higher medical education. *Am J Med Sci*. 1878; 76:174.

Billings JS. Commemoration of the one hundredth anniversary of the birth of, with various papers including two papers by Billings on medical education. *Bull Johns Hopkins Hosp*. 1938; 62:283.

Bonner TN. *Becoming a Physician: Medical Education in Britain, France, Germany, and the United States, 1750-1945*. Oxford: Oxford University Press; 1995.

Bordley J III, Harvey AM. *Two Centuries of American Medicine*. Philadelphia: W. B. Saunders; 1976.
Brown ER. *Rockefeller Medicine Men: Medicine and Capitalism in America*. Berkley: University of California Press; 1979.
Bynum WF. *Science and Practice of Medicine in the Nineteenth Century*. Cambridge: Cambridge University; 1994.
Carter BN. Fruition of Halsted's concept of surgical training. *Surgery*. 1952; 32:518.
Chesney AM. *The Johns Hopkins Hospital and the Johns Hopkins University School of Medicine*. 3 vol. Baltimore: Johns Hopkins; 1943, 1958, and 1963.
Crowe SJ. *Halsted of Johns Hopkins*. Springfield, Ill: Charles C. Thomas; 1957.
Cushing H. *The Life of Sir William Osler*. Oxford: Clarendon; 1926.
Davis AW. *Dr. Kelly of Hopkins*. Baltimore: Johns Hopkins; 1959.
Fleming D. *William H. Welch and the Rise of Modern Medicine*. Boston: Little and Brown; 1954.
Flexner A. *Medical Education in the United States and Canada*. New York: Carnegie Foundation for the Advancement of Teaching, No. 4; 1910.
French JC. *A History of the University Founded by Johns Hopkins*. Baltimore: Johns Hopkins; 1946.
Holman E. Sir William Osler and William Stewart Halsted – two contrasting personalities. *Pharos* 1971; 34:134.
Holman E. William Stewart Halsted. *Johns Hopkins Med J*. 1974; 135:418.
James H. *Charles W. Eliot, President of Harvard University, 1869-1909*. 2 vols. Boston and New York: Houghton Mifflin; 1930.
Ludmerer KM. *Learning to Heal: The Development of American Medical Education*. Boston: Basic Books; 1984.
-------- *Time to Heal: American Medical Education from the Turn of the Century to the Era of Managed Care*. Oxford: Oxford University Press; 1999.
MacCallum WG. *William Stewart Halsted*. Baltimore: Johns Hopkins; 1930.
Osler W. The inner history of the Johns Hopkins Hospital. Eds. DG Bates, EH Bensley. *Johns Hopkins Med J*. 1969; 125:184.
Rogers FB. *Selected Papers of John Shaw Billings, Compiled with a Life of Billings*. Chicago: Medical Library Association; 1965.
Roland GC et al. William Osler, 1849-1919 – commemorative issue. *JAMA* 1969; 210:2213-2271.
Sabin FR. *Franklin Pain Mall – The story of a Mind*. Baltimore: Johns Hopkins; 1934.
Shyrock RH. *Medical Licensing in American, 1650-1965*. Baltimore: Johns Hopkins; 1967.
Thom HH. *Johns Hopkins – Silhouette*. Baltimore: Johns Hopkins; 1929.
Thomas HM et al. Symposium on the development of the Johns Hopkins Medical School and Osler influence. *Bull Johns Hopkins Hosp*. 1919; 30:185.
Turner TB. *Heritage of Excellence*. Baltimore: Johns Hopkins; 1974.

Welch WH. Higher medical education and the need of its endowment. *Med News (Philadelphia)*. 1894; 65:63.
Welch WH. *Papers and Addresses*. 3 vols. Baltimore: Johns Hopkins; 1920.

Chapter 12: Modern Americans Arrive with More: The Twentieth Century Unfolds

Anton S. *Dates in Medicine: A Chronological Record of Medical Progress over Three Millennia.* New York: Parthenon Publishing; 2000.
Bonner TN. *Becoming a Physician: Medical Education in Britain, France, Germany, and the United States, 1750-1945.* New York: Oxford University Press; 1995
Bordley J III, Harvey AM. *Two Centuries of American Medicine.* Philadelphia: W. B. Saunders; 1976.
Brown ER. *Rockefeller Medicine Men: Medicine and Capitalism in America.* Berkley, CA: University of California Press; 1979.
Bynum WF. *Science and Practice of Medicine in the Nineteenth Century.* Cambridge: Cambridge University; 1994.
Cassedy JH. *Medicine in America: A Short History.* Baltimore: Johns Hopkins University Press; 1991.
Clendening L. Highlights of Twentieth Century Medicine. In: Ward H, ed. *New World's in Medicine: An Anthology.* New York: Robert M. McBride and Company; 1946.
Cut to the Heart: Pioneers of Heart Surgery. Nova Online. 1997. Available at: http://www.pbs.org/wgbh/nova/heart/pioneers.html
Duffin J. *History of Medicine: A Scandalously Short Introduction.* Toronto: University of Toronto Press; 1999.
Friedman M, Friedland G. *Medicine's 10 Greatest Discoveries.* New Haven: Yale University; 1998.
Gloub ES. *The Limits of Medicine: How Science Shapes our Hope for the Cure.* New York: Random House; 1994.
Leavitt JW and Numbers RL. *Sickness and Health in America.* Madison, WI: University of Wisconsin Press; 1985.
Ludmerer KM. *Time to Heal: American Medical Education from the Turn of the Century to the Era of Managed Care.* Oxford: Oxford University Press; 1999
MacKinnon B. *Human Cloning: Science, Ethics, and Public Policy.* Chicago: University of Illinois Press, 2000.
Medicine in the Postwar World. New York: Columbia University Press; 1948.
Reader's Digest, ed. *Milestones in Medicine.* New York: The Reader's Digest Association, Inc.; 1998.
Simmons JG. *Doctors and Discoveries: Lives that Created Today's Medicine.* Boston: Houghton Mifflin Co.; 2002.
Stevens R. *American Medicine and the Public Interest.* New Haven: Yale University; 1971.
Toledo-Pereyra LH. Harvey Cushing: Father of American Neurosurgery.

Journal of Investigative Surgery, 2002; 15:115-116.

-------- Visionary Mind of a Surgical Scientist: Marie Joseph Auguste Carrel. *Journal of Investigative Surgery*, 2002; 15:3-4.

-------- William Stewart Halsted: Father of American Modern Surgery. *Journal of Investigative Surgery*, 2002; 15:59-60.

Watson JD. *A Passion for DNA: Genes, Genomes, and Society*. Cold Spring Harbor, N.Y.: Cold Spring Harbor Laboratory Press; 2001.

INDEX